C

500
Excuses

&

500
Solutions

Tonna Brock, M.Ed, MS, LPC

For information contact:

Skinned Knees Publishing
P.O. Box 684, McKinney, Texas 75070
Telephone 972 837-5102
SkinnedKnees.com

First Edition

Cover design by Lionel Vera. Layout by Pam Posey.
Printed by Hignell Book Printing, LTD.,
Winnipeg, Manitoba, Canada

Library of Congress Control Number:
LCCN 2005909373

ISBN: 978-0-9774420-0-3

This book is dedicated to the loving memory of
Joan Copeland Voss (1931-1976)
and
Roger L. Voss (1949-2002).

Acknowledgements

Everyone I have had contact with in my life has helped weave the tapestry of my life. My gratitude overflows when I think of my life today. I would write another entire book if I start listing individuals. I thank my wonderful children Myka, Mekala, and Luke, who have grown up to be people I love having as friends. (Now, that is another entire book by itself.) They have sacrificed much and loved so well. I thank Wayne, my husband and dance partner, for listening to my ideas and being my sounding board. To my father, Lee and my wonderful other mother, Doris, I give thanks for their prayers, encouragement and love.

My family of choice has been so instrumental to my growth and development. They believed in me until I could believe in myself. My "sisters", my Wednesday meeting, my women's spirituality group, my colleagues, and my friends have always been there for me in the good, bad, happy, and sad times. You know who you are and where we have been together. May we continue this journey for a long, long time together.

My teachers have been many. I am grateful for all of my clients and students who shared their lives, pain, joy, and struggles with me and I wish them well. Through the years, I have crossed paths with so many interesting, loving people at retreats across America. I think of you often with warm memories.

I love the saying, "If you had fun, you won." I did and I have!

Tonna

Table of Contents

Side A – 500 Excuses

Side B – 500 Solutions

Introduction

This is a book of 500 Excuses and 500 Solutions for overeating. Which side you choose to read is your choice to make. It is not your mother's, father's, brother's, sister's, spouse's, friend's, medical doctor's, therapist's, nor anyone else's choice. It is yours.

I have met many overweight people in my personal life and career. I have met very few who wanted to be overweight. Most folks would choose to be of a normal size. "Just push away from the table" we have been told. We think, "Who needs a table?" We eat in the car, the bedroom, the living room, inside, outside, anywhere, everywhere; the time or place makes no difference. We eat and we eat.

According to the World Health Organization in the 2003 Obesity and Overweight Report, there are one billion overweight and 300 million obese people in the world. Most of us may not know how many, but we know it is a major health issue. The Centers for Disease Control and Prevention states the known health risks: hypertension, Dyslipemia (a big, fancy word for high total cholesterol or high levels of triglycerides), Type 2 diabetes, coronary heart disease, stroke, gallbladder disease, osteoarthritis, sleep apnea and respiratory problems. But still, we eat and we eat.

There was a drug that hit the market several years ago. It was supposed to create a "feeling of being full". Therefore, overweight folks would simply quit eating. We laughed. Did the scientists really think we stopped eating when full? Did they ever listen to what a fat person really was saying? We eat when we are so full that we think we will explode. That drug was taken off the market because of side effects that resulted in many deaths and permanent heart damage.

I do believe there are some overweight people who do not understand the concept of calories and exercise. If a person consumes more calories than she expends, she will gain weight. If he eats less than he burns, he will lose. Simple math. If someone eats or drinks 100 calories more than he needs every day for a year, he will gain over 10 pounds in a year. That is three-fourths of a can of soft drink, one tablespoon of regular salad dressing, or an extra teaspoon of margarine at each meal (100 X 365 =36,500 calories. There are 3500 calories in a pound.)

Then, the next year, it is ten more. After awhile, she decides to do something about it. Her medical doctor may hand her a "diet" or she goes to a dietician to learn how to eat healthy. She loses her excess weight and continues to closely monitor her weight. When she gains 3-5 pounds, she looks at where she is getting extra calories and reduces those or increases her exercise, thus losing the 3-5 pounds. This book may be helpful to those people.

However, I believe the majority of overweight people are compulsive overeaters. It is a disease. Food is a drug for them. Just as an alcoholic finds it nearly impossible to stop drinking, a compulsive overeater cannot stop eating. Oh, truthfully, we are great at stopping, especially on Monday and New Year's Day. We just cannot stay stopped.

Many of us have extensive knowledge about nutrition and exercise. Many of us have specialized in those areas, but to no avail. We are confused, frustrated, angry, sad, ashamed, embarrassed, humiliated, and frightened. We have tried countless ways and spent billions and billions of dollars, collectively, to lose weight and keep it off. There have been: bariatric physicians, diet clubs, herbal supplements, shots made from the urine of pregnant mares, speed, prescription and over the counter drugs, hypnosis, liquid protein, intestinal bypass, stomach stapling, stomach banding, liposuction, pre-packaged foods, jaws wired together, biofeedback, fasting, calorie counting, gyms, exercise equipment, low fat diets, low carb diets, clinic diets, high carb diets, diabetic diets, exchange diets, heart diets, endless magazine articles and hundreds of infomercials. Most of them worked, for a while.

According to the American Cancer Society the survival rates of over five years for many cancers are currently greater than 90%. Of people who lose weight, 98% regain it within five years!

Once, I was at a public meeting where a woman spoke of once weighing nearly 400 pounds and her subsequent recovery. A medical doctor, who is personal friend, made an interesting comment after hearing her. He said, "With all the money that could be made by drug companies, there will be a drug developed that will allow people to eat but not gain weight." I stood there wondering, what about the obsession? What about all the hours spent thinking about food, eating food, preparing food, waiting in lines to buy food, cooking food, going out to get food?

The weight is a symptom of the disease – not the disease. Is it not like saying, "let's use an effective drug to reduce fever, but let's not worry about treating the infection that is causing the fever?" Guess what, the fever will spike up once the fever medication is discontinued because the infection is worse. Just like weight (plus interest) is regained by simply going on a diet, unless the addiction is treated.

This book is not about articles or research about nutrition, obesity, overweight, exercise, statistics, empirical data, or the latest facts. You can look up those on the Internet or in a library. You can educate and entertain yourself for hours. That could be a noble goal, to learn more and more. I am leaving that search for you, if you are interested. I have found "knowing" wasn't my problem, it was "doing."

What are the reasons or causes of overeating? There are many. Most experts believe the cause is bio/psycho/social (biological, psychological, and social. What is not covered under that broad area, except it being a disease carried by UFO aliens?) We can all die of this while we try to figure out the cause. If we can stop, do we really care why we did it?

I promise you there is going to be nothing new or earth shattering in this book. Much of what you read here you may have already heard, read, or studied. I will try to give credit where credit is due. I've heard, but couldn't find the author of the quote, "All is wisdom plagiarized; only stupidity is original". There appears to be very few new ideas. Occasionally, I have come up with some brilliant, original concept. Then, I read it later in a book, written years before I came up with it. Drats, I hate that!

I admit I am prejudiced towards Twelve-Step programs. My personal recovery came as the result of working the steps. The steps originally come from Alcoholics Anonymous (AA). AA began when Bill W. met Dr. Bob in June 1935 in Akron, Ohio. According to a staff member at the General Services Office of Alcoholics Anonymous, as of December 2003, there have been 454 organizations that have been given permission to adapt the Twelve Steps[1] and Twelve Traditions[2] for their use. Obviously, I am not the only one who thinks they work!

Millions of people with all types of addictions, compulsions, diseases, issues, or problems have found recovery using the Steps and Traditions. We are all eternally grateful for the generous sharing of their program with other non-alcoholic organizations.

The purpose of this book is two-fold. It is to give you 500 Excuses and 500 Solutions for overeating. There are two lists, sometimes practical, sometimes ridiculous. It can be opened on any page and one or two ideas can be used. So, when you want to eat, there are 1000 things to read or do to not eat.

This is not a book written by someone who has just studied

the subject, but by me, who has lived it, personally. I began my journey of discovery and recovery 26 years ago. I am a Master's level licensed professional counselor so I have credentials and letters after my name. I started working in the eating disorder field over 17 years ago and have been in private practice for 13 years. However, most of my wisdom has come from skinned knees and elbows.

My intent is to write this book like I am talking to my reader. I have put inner-thoughts in parentheses because that is the way I talk. Sometimes, I take the scenic tour to tell a simple story. I will try to refrain from using multiple "!!!!!!!!" but that is how passionate I get about many things.

I watched my mother and brother die from overeating. I want to do whatever I can to prevent another compulsive overeater's death. My hopes are that this book will give you ideas to help you develop a lifestyle instead of continuing to live a "deathstyle".

As you will notice, there are actually two books you are holding. 500 Excuses and 500 Solutions. You decide which one you want to read. If you start in the 500 Excuses, you are the one who will have to turn it around to read the solutions. You can stay in the Excuses.

I had to *do* something different to *get* something different. I learned that, if everyday I went home and made my brownie recipe when I opened the oven door, there would be a pan of brownies. I could not make the recipe and expect there to be a pan of cornbread when I opened the door. If I wanted to make cornbread, I would use some of the same ingredients but have to change some of them. If I want things to be different in my life, I have to change some of the things I am doing. For me, not making my brownie *or* cornbread recipe was a start.

500 Excuses or 500 Solutions.   It is your choice.

[1]The Twelve Steps of Alcoholics Anonymous

1. We admitted we were powerless over alcohol- that our lives had become unmanageable.

2. Came to believe that a Power greater than ourselves could restore us to sanity.

3. Made a decision to turn our will and our lives over to the care of God as *we understood Him.*

4. Made a searching and fearless inventory of ourselves.

5. Admitted to God, to ourselves, and to another human being the exact nature of our wrongs.

6. Were entirely ready to have God remove all these defects of character.

7. Humbly asked Him to remove our shortcomings.

8. Made a list of all persons we had harmed, and became willing to make amends to them all.

9. Made direct amends to such people wherever possible, except when to do so would injure them or others.

10. Continued to take personal inventory and when we were wrong, promptly admitted it.

11. Sought through prayer and meditation to improve our conscious contact with God *as we understand Him,* praying only for knowledge of His will for us and the power to carry that out.

12. Having had a spiritual awakening as the result of these steps, we tried to carry this message to alcoholics, and practice these principles in all of our affairs.

[2]The Twelve Traditions of Alcoholics Anonymous

One – Our common welfare should come first: personal recovery depends upon A.A. Unity.

Two – For our group purpose there is but one ultimate authority – a loving God as He may express Himself in our group conscience. Our leaders are but trusted servants: they do not govern.

Three – The only requirement for A.A. membership is a desire to stop drinking.

Four – Each group should be autonomous except in matters affecting A.A. as a whole.

Five – Each group has but one primary purpose – to carry its message to the alcoholic who still suffers.

Six – An A.A. group ought never endorse, finance, or lend the A.A. name to any related facility or outside enterprise, lest problems of money, property and prestige divert us from our primary purpose.

Seven – Every A.A. group ought to be fully self-supporting, declining outside contributions.

Eight – Alcoholics Anonymous should remain forever nonprofessional, but our service centers may employ special workers.

Nine – A.A., as such, ought never be organized: but we may create service boards directly responsible to those they serve.

Ten – Alcoholics Anonymous has no opinions on outside issues; hence the A.A. name ought never be drawn into public controversy.

Eleven – Our public relations policy is based on attraction rather than promotion; we need to always maintain personal anonymity at the level of press, radio, and films.

Twelve – Anonymity is the spiritual foundation of all of our Traditions, ever reminding us to place principles before personalities.

Chapter One

A Day in the Life of a Compulsive Overeater

7:00 AM:
Surely it can't be morning already. I'm going to just lie here five more minutes. What am I going to make for Alex for breakfast? Today's the day. Today I **have** to stay on my diet. I feel terrible. I feel nauseated.[3] I wish I could stay in bed all day, just pull up the covers and ignore the world and all its demands on me.

It's only eight weeks until Carol's wedding and I **have** to lose these fifty pounds.[11] I really love Carol and I can't let her down, but there is no way I can go home and let all of my friends see me like this.[8] I wonder if Kenneth will be there. I would die if he saw me looking like this.

I can't believe I have gained fifty pounds in these last 10 years. Boy, that's a joke! I've gained hundreds of pounds. I lost 20 on the starvation soup diet, 14 on the ski diet,[9] 10 in the wiener, egg, and banana diet, and, of course, I lost those 46 when I was going to the diet doctor.[14] That was the easiest way, those wonderful magic pills, no hunger, plenty of energy, my house got clean, and the weight fell off! I know Rick and I would be divorced if I had kept taking them. I couldn't control myself. I was so irritable all the time; I had rages, and forget about sleep unless I took sleeping pills to bring me down. I think Beth must be on them. She is losing weight and she seems so nervous lately. I might call her later to find out where she is getting them.

Today I am going to just eat a piece of toast for breakfast with black coffee. I have just **got** to do this. I have done it in the past and I can do it again.

7:20 AM:
Oh, no, if I don't hurry Alex will be late for school again. Why did I stay in bed so long? Oops, I forgot when I took that

bite out of Alex's leftover donut, but I spit it out so it doesn't count. I had best get it out of the trashcan and put it down the disposal. I hate it when I stay in bed and then I yell at Alex to hurry. I wish he could leave happy from the house in the morning. I wish I could be a better mother. I really do love him, Becky, and Rick. I am so lucky to have such a precious family and live in this nice home. Why am I so miserable? What more could I possibly want out of life?

10:00 AM:
I guess it's safe for me to eat my toast now. I feel faint. My blood sugar may be dropping. Becky is driving me crazy. She has whined and cried all morning. Thank God for morning naps!

I should exercise while Becky's out of my hair. Let's see, what program will I do? I'll do the aerobic video for 40 minutes, that's pretty hard. I should try to jog 3 miles at least 5 days a week or ride my stationary bicycle 45 minutes a day. Oh, I can't remember which one burns up the most calories. I'll go look it up.

Oh, my gosh, look at all these diet, exercise books, and videos I have in this closet. I've got a better selection and as many different ones as Roy's Bookstore does. Some of these are so out of date. I didn't realize how quickly these fads come and go. Here is the number one bestseller from 1995. I haven't heard anyone mention it in ages. Hey, this low-carb is making another comeback so I may need to re-read it tomorrow. Each one of these is "The Last Diet Book You Will Ever Need To Buy".

I really should throw some of these away. Rick would be so upset if he finds all of these and adds up how much I have spent on them. Just add that to his complaining about not having room in the garage because of all the exercise equipment I have accumulated through the years! He wanted me to sell them in the garage sale but I am still planning on using them.

When I think of the money I have spent on diets, diet doctors, spas, hypnosis, diet books, shots, pills, gyms, weight loss clinics, and exercise equipment, it's so depressing. I could have traveled around the world on what I have spent already.

I wish there was a way to just take an exam and get a degree for exercise, nutrition and weight counseling. I would have a PHD. I am a smart, intelligent woman. Why, why, if I know so much, do I have so much trouble doing it?

11:30 AM
I can't believe Rick just called and he wants to go out to eat tonight with the Blackwells. He knows I can't stand Jill. I don't know what I will wear. I guess my blue denim dress. It doesn't look too much like a maternity dress. I could go shopping after we pick up Alex from school, but I hate to spend any money on this size clothes. I really want to find the slinkiest, sexiest outfit for Carol's wedding. I want to make all my old friends jealous.

I better not eat lunch today since we are going out to eat tonight. I'll just save my calories for then. Rick should have been more considerate of me. He knew I was starting on my diet today. I could lose weight easier if he supported me more. I hate him when he smarts off like he did on the phone. I begged him not to make us go tonight, of all nights. He said that I start a diet every Monday morning. Even if it is true, he didn't have to say it.[10] This time it is different. I have to do it.

12:15 PM
Becky, please eat all of your sandwich. I need to eat something. I'm starving, but I need to save my calories. I guess I'll have a bouillon cube in hot water, that's supposed to help fill you up. Of course, the extra sodium may cause me to retain water so I will take a diuretic, too. Oh, I nearly forgot to start drinking 10 glasses of water a day. I'll just finish Becky's apple. Maybe I will eat the rest of her

sandwich. No, no, I won't. I really need something to tide me over. It's not really that much.⁴ I've got to put the chips down the disposal. I think I'll take Becky for a walk. Anything to get me out of the kitchen. They wouldn't put an alcoholic in a bar all day. I better call and try to get a sitter for tonight. Rick always makes these decisions and then I am stuck phoning all day trying to find someone. It is just not worth it. I wish I could stay home tonight.

3:15 PM

I can't believe that I am in the kitchen again! Alex is getting old enough to get his own snack, but he makes such a mess. I know I could lose weight if I didn't have to feed these kids. If I was single like Carol, I would be thin as a model. Food, food, food, all day long. I have to plan, shop, prepare, and clean-up, constantly. Before the kids came, I wasn't much better but I was under so much stress from my teaching job. Why is every commercial on television this afternoon about candy, cereal, junk, and fast food?¹² I'll get the kids some cookies as soon as I am stronger, but until I have a few days on my diet, I can't have it in the house. It's probably not that good for them either. Alex is getting chunky already. God, please don't let him be a fat child. I know what a hell it is to be the fat kid at school. I will never get over that nightmare I lived. Kids are so cruel to each other.

5:15 PM

I think I better go eat something. Rick will pick me up in another hour and we won't eat for at least two hours. If I eat something now, I will be able to eat moderately tonight. I'll only have white wine because the daiquiris are loaded with sugar. I'll eat this frozen diet dinner. This makes a total of 487 calories so far today. I think I will let the sitter feed the kids.

6:30 PM

I know Rick is embarrassed about his business friends seeing his fat, ugly cow still in her maternity clothes and Becky is 18 months old. Oh, look at Jill in that tank top and tight designer jeans. I bet she had to lie down on the bed to zip them up. She looks like a call girl. Why can't she dress her age? I wonder if she has stretch marks on her stomach or if she is firm and tan all over. She probably sunbathes in a skimpy swimsuit with her "store bought" breasts hanging out. She is so thin. I bet she pukes. Just for spite, I might go to the ladies' room with her after dinner so she can't purge tonight. Look at her laughing and acting so cute. She makes me so sick.

I'll just order a chef salad.[7] I want to eat the chips and cheese queso. I'll get a breath mint so my mouth is busy. I can't start on the chips because I can't stop after a couple. They ordered loaded baked potatoes, steak, and sourdough bread. How many calories in that! No, I'll stick with the salad. I'll eat three packs of crackers, no, two. I'll wait and see if two are enough. Look at how much Jill left on her plate. When I lose all of my weight, I'll start leaving half of my food on my plate and I will probably be able to maintain.

I should ask for a doggie bag for Rick's leftovers. That's appropriate because I am the dog that eats them and I look like a dog. No, I can't trust myself yet. I shouldn't have those last two packages of crackers. I should have stopped with three, but I didn't use all of my salad dressing.

Please, no, please help me! They are all ordering cheesecake with raspberries and chocolate sauce. Look at how smooth and creamy it is. I love the New York style and that is what it looks like. I'll ask Rick for a taste, just one tiny, lousy bite. That look of disgust in Rick's eyes cuts me to the core; he really doesn't need to ever say anything. Thank goodness, he doesn't say a word to me in public about my weight or my food, but those looks.[10] Oh, that is so good! I wonder if it is always this good? As soon as I get off this diet, I am coming back here alone and eat all of that cheesecake I can, to heck with the dinners.[5] Jill only ate four bites of hers. I would almost kill for it and she is leaving those plump, juicy berries and that cool, smooth, sweet,

14

creamy cake. I wonder if they use vanilla wafers or graham crackers for a crust. I might make that low-cal cheesecake recipe with the sugarless cookies tomorrow. I could have a small slice for breakfast and two for lunch and two for dinner and nothing else.

Robert makes me sick. He is so affectionate in public. Look at the way Robert and Jill smile dreamily like they can't get enough of each other. They have been married even longer than we have and they act like newlyweds. I'm so thankful we are finally leaving. I'm about to scream.

10:15 PM
I'll go ahead and get ready for bed while Rick drives the sitter home. This kitchen is trashed. I can't believe they wasted almost a whole bag of chips. I'll clean this up first. I won't eat but this one handful.[13] There can't be that many calories in this small amount.

I am so angry at Rick! He took up for Robert and Jill on the way home. I can't believe he thinks Jill looks good, the way she flaunts her body. Surely, he can see she is as plastic as a credit card. I don't know why Rick and I are always bickering lately.I am so tired. I'm proud of how well I did with my food today. I should have done better but it wasn't too bad under the circumstances.

11:05 PM
If I turn my back on Rick, maybe he won't start anything tonight. He's snuggling. Should I turn over? Oh, God, he just touched my belly. Why can't he just touch my face? I can't stand his hands rubbing over my rolls of fat. Don't let me stiffen up. It's not that I don't want him, but I can't tolerate myself. I wonder who he imagines I am when he makes love to me? He has to have a great imagination or he could never force himself to touch this body of blubber. I'll go ahead and have sex because that is the least I can do.

He is such a great guy. I feel so bad because I played

such a perfect part while we were dating. He thought I was wonderful, sweet, adoring. Little did he know the real me, but I did. I knew I could not control the swings in my weight except for occasions like Carol's wedding. I have lived this nightmare since I was 9 years old.

11:30 PM

I can't go to sleep. How many nights have I listened until Rick's breathing became even? I think I will get up and read. It is useless to just lay here.

I think I'll look in the refrigerator to see what I can cook tomorrow. That cheesecake does sound good. I'd forgotten about this old gelatin salad in this container. I'll eat it since it won't be any good tomorrow. I wonder why old gelatin gets so tough on top. What's this? Cold pizza. What would I do without a microwave?

I wonder if there is any candy around. I need something sweet. I threw away all that was in the candy dishes last night. I need to get this taste out of my mouth. Maybe there are some mints in my purse. No such luck! I wonder if Alex has any more candy in his jack-o'-lantern. I know I ate all the chocolate the night he got home. I'll sneak into his closet and check. I can't believe this, not even any in the drawer under the sheets in the guest room.[6]

Do I dare leave and go through the 24 hour donut shop drive-thru? Rick would freak out if he woke up and I wasn't here. I'm not that brave, but I need something. I know, cinnamon toast! Thank goodness for frozen bread. I wish I had one of those frozen cakes with the chocolate icing. I wonder what they taste like after thawing. I've always eaten them frozen. I ate that can of frosting last night and it was the last one in the pantry.

I'd better close the bedroom door. Hopefully, Rick won't smell the toast cooking. Funny, in these past 10 years, he has only caught me that one time when Alex had a bad dream. Should I make three pieces? No, I'll make six. I can heat the leftovers in the morning for the kids. No, I'll make them some fresh. I'll just eat these since I hate to throw out good food. I love the taste of butter melted into the soft bread and the crunch of the sugar when it is broiled. It is just like my mother made me as a child.

1:30 AM
I've done it again! Should I figure up all the calories I ate today? Oh, what is the use? I'll start tomorrow. I should have known I couldn't stay on my diet if we went out tonight. I wish I had a piece of that delicious cheesecake. I hate me.[15] Am I crazy? I wish I could die. I wish I had the guts to end this insanity. I can't hurt my children that way. It would be taking all of my pain and giving it to them. I'd probably go to Hell. My luck, Hell would be me, surrounded by all of my favorite foods for all of eternity and not being able to eat a bite.

I'll **have** to stay on my diet tomorrow. Carol's wedding is coming. I hurt. I feel so bloated and swollen. Will my stomach burst someday?[1] If only I had some willpower. If only I didn't have to spend so much time in the kitchen. If only I lived alone, if only, if only!

I will do it. I can do it. Didn't I stay on that diet for six weeks last June? Maybe, I'll call that doctor that gives those shots, just to give me a little head start. I might be able to cut back on spending at the grocery store so Rick won't know. Heck, no binges will save us a fortune!

I promise I **will not** overeat tomorrow. Sure, I said that last night, but tonight I **really** mean it. Why? Why me, God? I hate me.

I wonder what color dress I should buy for the wedding. I think royal blue or hot pink. It has to have sleeves. I think my silver sandals will look good with either color.

2:00 AM
I've got to find the liquid antacid. I ate all the tablets last week. My heartburn is terrible. Oh, no, it's so late. What was I thinking? I've got to get some sleep!

The superscript numbers correspond with the 15 Questions
Copyright © Overeaters Anonymous.

Are You A Compulsive Overeater?

This series of questions may help you determine if you are a compulsive overeater. Many members of Overeaters Anonymous have found that they have answered yes to many of these questions.

1. Do you eat when you're not hungry?
2. Do you go on eating binges for no apparent reason?
3. Do you have feelings of guilt and remorse after overeating?
4. Do you give too much time and thought to food?
5. Do you look forward with pleasure and anticipation to the time when you can eat alone?
6. Do you plan these secret binges ahead of time?
7. Do you eat sensibly before others and make up for it alone?
8. Is your weight affecting the way you live your life?
9. Have you tried to diet for a week (or longer), only to fall short of your goal?
10. Do you resent others telling you to "use a little willpower" to stop overeating?
11. Despite evidence to the contrary, have you continued to assert that you can diet "on your own" whenever you wish?
12. Do you crave to eat at a definite time, day or night, other than mealtime?
13. Do you eat to escape from worries or trouble?
14. Have you ever been treated for obesity or a food related condition?
15. Does your eating behavior make you or others unhappy?

Have you answered yes to three or more of these questions? If so, it is probable that you have or are well on the way to having a compulsive overeating problem. We have found that the way to arrest this progressive disease is to practice the twelve-step recovery program of Overeaters Anonymous.

Chapter Two

My Story – The Disease

I was born at a very early age into a family with eating issues. To understand where I developed some of my crazy food behaviors, I will explain some of what I watched, heard, and learned as a child. I had a professor in graduate school who had us write papers on our childhood. Someone asked what to do if we did not remember our childhood. He said, "Make it up, because we make it all up anyhow." This is my perception of my family and my life as seen through my eyes. It may not be reality.

Great-Grandparents

I remember my great-grandmother being very overweight. She sat listening to the radio and doing needlework. I never saw her get up very much. She was known for her pies. Because she didn't have many pie pans, sometimes she would stack several sweet potato pies up on top of each other and then cut them like a layered cake. As a small child, I was always fascinated by the sight of my great-grandfather's glasses of iced tea with half the glass full of sugar and a whole lemon. I never saw him stir it up.

Grannie

My Grannie, my maternal grandmother, and I were very close. Probably, because we had a common enemy, my parents. (Just joking.) She was 34 years old when my brother was born and 36 when I came along. She lived across the street from me and I went to play with her for hours. She would bathe me, wash my hair and clothes. She would mop her floors and clean her oven very fast and often. This was assisted by the 17 diet pills, the black Mollies, she took a day. She had started taking them one a day and when that lost effectiveness, she took 2, then 3, then 4 until she hit 17 a day.

Eventually, she had to go to a mental hospital because of her bizarre behavior and the fact that she didn't sleep for weeks. The medical professionals at the hospital took her off the diet pills. Her local MD wrote her more prescriptions. I remember sitting in the car with Grannie while my 5-year-old brother, Roger, would take the empty bottle into the pharmacy and come out with another bottle. Once Grannie complained that mother would borrow diet pills, not to try to lose weight but because she needed to clean house.

I was 9 years old the first time I ever saw my Grannie eat at a regular mealtime. My Dad had grilled steaks. I ran around all excited because she was eating! She drank a coffee in the morning with a few ginger snaps. I don't remember seeing her very often during the day without a soft drink in her lap. About one o'clock in the morning she would cook homemade corn dogs (she had mastered her own recipe), frozen hushpuppies, pickles and sliced tomatoes. I asked her why she only ate in the middle of the night. She told me that when she ate her stomach swelled.

Before eating, she took about 3 doses each of 3 different laxatives. I asked, "Why do you take so many laxatives?" She told me she had a small colon and couldn't go to the bathroom without them. When Grannie was 62, she went to a specialist who told her she had to get off all the laxatives. She said she couldn't have bowel movements without them. He said, "Eat bran cereal." She did and she could! The whole family was so excited when Grannie had a natural BM.

A few months later, she came for a visit and she was taking all of her laxatives again. I asked her "Why?" She said, "Honey, I was getting so fat I couldn't fit into my wheelchair." That's when I knew. She had been using them to purge all those years and that is what caused her swollen stomach. (I would have tried laxatives, too but I could never figure how to manage the diarrhea and my busy lifestyle.)

Grannie always took many, many pills. I would pray every night from a very early age that God wouldn't let her die. Once, she threw a huge bottle of pills at my cousin when he smart-mouthed her when he was seven. He told her, "That's what I like about you, Grannie. You have spunk". She did have a wonderful sense of humor and played tricks on everyone. She entertained me for hours with her stories.

Her MD told her to stop smoking if she wanted to live longer. She told him, "Who wants to live longer if I can't smoke?" Grannie was diagnosed with Type 2 diabetes and put on insulin. Within a month, she had a heart attack and died at the age of 70.

Mother

Momma got married when she was 17 and my father was 22. Daddy worked at a lumberyard and threw 100 pound bags of cement off of rail cars and had big rocks for muscles. Momma said the first meal she cooked was 5 slices of bacon, 3 for him and 2 for her, macaroni and cheese, and sliced tomatoes. She said Daddy told her, "This isn't enough food. I'll bring home the bacon and you put it on table." He did and she did.

Both parents were great cooks. We ate wonderful chicken-fried steak, mashed potatoes, gravy and biscuits, cakes, pies, cookies, fried catfish, homemade hushpuppies, hot German potato salad, fried egg sandwiches. Lots of food and lots of love were always available at my house.

I remember my brother's friend coming to dinner one night when I was in the second grade. He was so amazed at the fact we could eat all we wanted. He lived in a big, white, two-storied house. His mother was thin and beautiful. His family looked like one of the perfect ones I saw on television. She made one serving of meat for each person and brought it to the table on individual plates, not heaping platters. I think he got sick that night from eating so much. That was the first time I learned other families didn't eat like mine. He loved coming to our house to visit.

Momma said she started gaining weight after she got pregnant. Roger was born when she was 18. The doctor told her if she didn't lose weight, she was going to have diabetes, cancer, heart problems, gallbladder, arthritis and other health issues. She didn't like being told that on every doctor visit. She just stopped going to the doctor.

I was emotionally torn when I started to school. I loved my mother so very much and I was also embarrassed because she was fat. The other children would tell me my mother was fat as if I didn't know. I felt guilty for being embarrassed.

Mother joined some diet group. She dyed long knee length underwear and tee shirts black to do exercise in. After her class, they went to the bowling alley for chef salads. Once she found a diet doctor who gave her about ten different colored pills. They came from his office, not a pharmacy. She had to take them at different times of the day. She kept them in a coffee can.

In her twenties, Momma had arthritis and took cortisone for relief. She stopped menstruating when she was about 29. One day, she mentioned to a friend that she hadn't had a period in about four years. Her friend invited her to lunch the next week. When she picked Mother up, she told her that first my mother had an appointment with a gynecologist.

He could tell by visual examination that she had cervical cancer. She was to go immediately to the hospital. She had radium and cobalt treatments. Because of the radiation, she was in a special room in the hospital and we could only spend a few minutes with her each day. I spent my thirteenth birthday eating out with Daddy after visiting my mother in the hospital.

My paternal grandmother, Ma, had stomach cancer at the same time. I heard she was dying. My mother had cancer. I was told not to tell Grannie about some of mother's medical issues because my mother didn't want her to worry. I didn't tell and I did the worrying.

Two years later, at the age of 35 my mother was diagnosed with diabetes. She was to take insulin shots in the morning. The first day out of the hospital, there was a mix-up on the strength and amount she was supposed to take. She started shaking and having an insulin reaction. She called her doctor's office and was told to eat six candy bars as fast as she could. She came home from work and said, "You know, I bet I could take two shots on Thanksgiving and eat whatever I want." She would eat correctly in the morning and binge on sugar at night. I would go with her to get ice cream bars at the convenience store. I worried about her, but I liked the sweet treats.

My mother suffered a heart attack when she was 38 years old. The new doctor told her she never should have been put on insulin. She should have been controlling her insulin levels with her diet. She was put on a 400 calorie per day diet. I think she got to smell toast for breakfast! She started losing weight and I was so proud of her. She said she would soon be able to wear my clothes. I wanted her to be thin, but not thinner than me. I felt so guilty and ashamed for feeling that way.

Momma was about 39 when she had to be rushed to the hospital with what we thought was another heart attack. It was a gallbladder attack. She said the symptoms felt the very same.

My mother was one of the funniest people I've ever met. She never met a stranger and was so much fun! My house was **THE** hangout for my high-school years. I never remember a night when there were not kids over visiting. That was a blessing and a curse at the same time. My friends would come confide in her when they broke up with their girlfriends or boyfriends. My mother was greatly loved by so many.

At 43 years of age, my mother was told her cancer had returned after 10 years of remission and she had six months to a year to live. She lived two years, if you want to call it living. Watching a loved one, vibrant and so full of life, physically rot away from cancer, has got to be Hell on earth. She was in excruciating pain almost constantly. I don't know whose pain was worse, hers or ours watching her suffer.

I was very dependent on my mother. We were too close, enmeshed in many ways. She lived her life through mine. Today, I can see how unhealthy our relationship was; however, I don't think I would change much about it. While she was dying she said, "Some people have their mothers until they are 90 and never get along. We have had such a short time, but it has been quality." She really knew how to keep the fun in dys<u>fun</u>ctional.

On a hot, dusty day in July, we buried my mother. Forty-five short years. Twenty-five years earlier, her doctor had told her she would have cancer, diabetes, heart problems, arthritis, and gallbladder attacks. She did.

Father

My father overate at meals but did not appear to have the compulsive eating patterns of other family members. He was 30-35 pounds overweight, but nothing very noticeable for his height. A year and a half after my mother's death, Daddy had open-heart surgery with seven bypasses done on his arteries. He was 51 years old and a walking candidate for a coronary. At age 65, he had to have four of them redone. He has been on medication for hypertension for over 20 years. At 67, he had to have his gallbladder removed. Dad had prostate cancer when he was 74. He has sixty percent blockage of the carotid artery.

My father and mother taught me love is an action verb. They loved people and had many friends of different cultures. Our home was always open. My father and other mother are actively involved in helping others. Lately, there have been several homeless people they have been taking to lunch and helping to find clothing. I was taught the three r's - respect, responsibility, and reliability.

Recently, my husband said my father spoiled me. When I laughingly shared that comment with my father, he said, "He's got the wrong word, it's loved, not spoiled." I'm the first to admit my Daddy spoiled and loved me.

Brother

Roger was two and a half years older than I. He was my only sibling. He was always heavy in my memories except for the old photos when he was about two years old. He was good in sports even though being overweight. We moved when he was in the fifth grade. The Little League teams were fourth, fifth, and sixth graders. He was drafted as a new member. The first game, he did not play. My mother called the coach and asked "why not?" He told her it was because my brother was too fat to play baseball. I was seven years old when I heard my mother tell this story. I was shocked his coach would tell a fat mother that her son was too fat! She told him to give him a chance. He made the All-Star team that year.

Roger was a smoker, overweight and a successful, hardworking, Type A personality. One Christmas when we were celebrating at my house, he told my son, "Come down to our house where you can eat real food, not all this fat-free shit."

He had his first heart attack when he was 42 years old. I got the phone call from my sister-in law in the early morning hours. She was distraught. She asked me to call my father's hospital, where he was recovering from his second set of bypasses, to see if he was stable enough for me to tell him about my brother.

Roger was in intensive care for almost a month. One night, I got a call that his heart had stopped and I needed to get to the hospital ASAP. The medical staff was able to revive him. Eventually, his cardiologist was able to do bypass surgery. Eighty percent of his heart was damaged, but the bypass was successful. The next Christmas, at his house, we all ate fat-free mayo and fat-free cheese.

In the Spring of 2002, Roger's feet were swelling and he was on very expensive medications because only twenty percent of his heart was working, even though he was still giving two hundred percent at his job. His company had received "vendor of the year" from a major do-it-yourself retail store chain due to his hard work. I asked him why he did not get a heart transplant. He said he wasn't a candidate because he was obese. Six weeks later, he had a fatal heart attack at the age of 53.

Me

Pre-school Years

The stories I heard as a little girl affected me for a long time. I was told my mother didn't want to be pregnant with me. She didn't have good rhythm. I didn't feel wanted. My Dad reportedly was happy because he wanted a blonde-haired, blue-eyed, baby girl. I was, until second grade when my hair turned brown, my eyes green, and I got fat. Guess what I believed?

My Grannie told me that she loved me and I was her favorite. She told me my great-grandmother and other grandmother didn't like me. It was really obvious that my brother was loved better by them. I grew up feeling I had to "make" people like and love me. I wasn't lovable, just because.

Grannie said that she had been spanked very hard as a child and my parents would have to fight with her in order to discipline us when she was around. We lived across the street from her. One day, when I was three, I was over there playing tea party with her. My father came to pick me up and take me home. I, immediately, ran back across the street. One of my parents came and got me and spanked my bottom. I went to bed sobbing, "I want, I want my Ga.. Ga...*Gannie*." Grannie was heartbroken I got a spanking and I was begging for her. She was scared that I would get hit by a car while running over to her house.

The next time I was over, she told me, "That won't work. When your Daddy comes to get you, run up to him, tell him how much you love him and are so happy to see him. That way they will let you come back." I was three years old and was being taught to deny what I really wanted, be dishonest, and to manipulate men! It seems so interesting how such seemingly innocent incidents have such long lasting effects on children.

Elementary School

I first recall my weight in the first grade. The school nurse came and weighed us. I weighed 56 pounds and the girl who lived behind us weighed 27. I had a 28-inch waist in the second grade. Today, I think how bizarre it is that I remember my weight at that early age.

Whenever I was sick, my mother would get me anything I wanted to eat. I usually ordered fried shrimp. Even when I had a stomach virus, I ate fried shrimp from the drive-in restaurant. I had it and Texas toast the day after I had my tonsils removed. That wasn't a wise choice on my part.

When I was in the second grade, my parents were having a fight and I was afraid they would get a divorce. I felt my whole world was collapsing. Some friends came over during it and we all acted as if nothing was going on. I watched my parents laugh and joke with them. After they left, we had dinner very late as we normally ate dinner at 5:15 every night. My parents put my brother and me to bed so we could go to school the next morning. When Momma woke me up, she said it was not what we had thought the night before. She told me a lie. Years later, my brother laughed at me for believing the story. I still believed in Santa Claus so why wouldn't I believe my mother? I learned some powerful lessons that day that took years to unlearn. No matter what is going on, don't let anyone know. If you eat and go to sleep, when you wake up, everything is going to be good again. No matter what, lie your way out of it.

We had moved to a new school and a new town in October of my second grade. My report card stated my comprehension was better than my oral reading. That was because I hated reading out loud. I would call "and" "the" and "it" "but". I was afraid of making a "public" mistake in reading circle. I was placed in the "slow-learners" class. After a few days, the teacher knew that was a mistake. The school staff felt it was better for me to remain in that class than to switch again. The teacher sent me to the library most of the day to read. Read, I did. I read a lot. Reading became a major escape for me for many years. When I was reading, I wasn't facing the realities of my life. I could eat a bag of lemon drops and stay in my room and read. Eating and reading were my best friends.

In the third grade, my mother got me diet pills from her friend whose husband was a pharmaceutical rep. They would get them from his big black case when he was playing golf. I think they just made me eat faster.

I was placed in the "accelerated" class in the third grade. Those kids were real smart and knew the names of every dinosaur. By the fourth grade, I was so nervous about test taking, my stomach would cramp so much. I was prescribed "nerve" medication.

In the fourth grade when the nurse weighed me, I was 114 pounds. There was only one other kid who weighed over 100 pounds, just the fat boy. She called the weight out loud to someone who recorded it. I'll never forget the shocked whispers of my classmates, "Gosh, she weighs over 100". I just wanted the floor to open up and swallow me.

I went to the movies nearly every week as a child. They had the saltiest popcorn in the world. I had to have a soft drink with it. The fountain soft drinks were the sweetest in the world. I had to have something salty with it, like their popcorn. I believe that is where I developed that sweet/salt craving. I had to have something salty after something sweet. Then, I had to have something sweet after the salt. People would talk about something being too rich. I never understood what that meant. One day it hit me! Of course, that is when the icing was so sweet that I had to have mixed nuts with it.

The movie theatre had discounted tickets for those under twelve. The lady would question me and give me looks when I would ask for a child's ticket. My mother started sending my birth certificate to the movies with me. I hated being big and fat. Sometimes, I wondered if I my mother had kept me in a closet and let me out when I was three and told me I was a newborn.

One day, a boy called me "fatty" and made fun of me on the way home from school. I ignored him. I was good at ignoring because I had an older brother who teased me most of the time, it seemed. The next day the principal came over the loud speaker at school and asked the teacher to send me to the office. There was the boy and the principal made him apologize to me because someone had told on him. I wanted to die. Now the principal knew! When I got back to my classroom, my classmates wanted to know if I was in trouble. I really wanted to die.

Being a fat kid is one of the most horrible nightmares a child has to endure. My self-concept will possibly always be as a fat person, no matter what the scale says.

I cried alone and wondered why I was left out when God was giving talents. Many of my friends were good at singing, sports, art, or music. I was uncoordinated and tone deaf. My mother actually paid me to not practice the violin. I felt good at nothing. I was bigger than my fourth grade teacher. I was 5'2". I felt so fat, ugly, and hopeless. (I haven't grown in height since sixth grade. I am still 5'4".) One day in college, I ran into a former classmate from elementary school, she looked down at me and said, "What happened to you? You were a giant.")

Honestly, in the fifth grade I went to a carnival at the shopping center by my house. After getting off a ride, I noticed a very petite classmate and her tiny sister. I waited on them to get off the ride so I could talk to them. The ride operator asked me if they were my kids. I was eleven years old. I almost died from shock and embarrassment.

I took ballroom dancing lessons. We did a special dance demonstration one evening at a local club. At practice, there was the very cutest boy I'd ever seen. He was dancing with the cheerleader who was so pretty. My partner never spoke to me, or for that matter, probably never even looked at me. The night of the performance, the cheerleader wore high-heels which made her taller than me. We were switched and I danced with the dreamy guy. Instead of being thrilled, I felt sorry for him. He was stuck with me.

Junior High

We had a new house built in a different school district when I was in the seventh grade. The school was much smaller, in the suburbs. School started and Momma was diagnosed with cancer the same month. Many of the kids had been together since first grade. I was the fat, ugly, new girl. I cried myself to sleep more nights than I want to remember.

I babysat the neighbor's children. I would start eating ice cream and be embarrassed by how much I ate. It came in a cardboard brick. Sometimes, I took out a few scoops from the bottom of the container so it wouldn't look like I ate as much as I did.

By the eighth grade, Mother's cancer was in remission and I became her new mission. She was determined to "make" me popular. She started having slumber parties for me. Between the eighth and ninth grade, I went on a diet. I froze a can of liquid diet drink and ate it. The directions said to drink four cans a day. There were 800 calories. I was good at math. Therefore, if I could lose weight on 800 calories, what could I do on 200! I allowed myself one stick of chewing gum and walked six miles a day. I lost about twenty pounds in a month. I got so much praise! My mother was so pleased. Today, it would be called anorexia.

High School

Ninth grade was like a fairy tale come true. I was living the "Ugly Duckling" story. Many of the boys who had hated me were asking me out. Sometimes, I wanted them to fall madly in love with me as sweet revenge for how they treated me the previous years. I majored in "boyology". I usually ate one third of a sandwich with my friends at lunch so we could get to the gym to flirt with the senior boys. As soon as I found one I was attracted to, I would stop eating because I wanted to be thinner. After I lost attraction for him, I would eat again. Today I realize those wonderful, funny feelings of "love" I felt in my stomach were really hunger pangs. I fell "in" and "out" of love pretty often that freshman year.

My house was the place to be in high school. I had so many friends. It was such a good time. I am still friends with many of them. We all agree that those were the days. My class has reunions every five years. The class behind me has yet to have one. I talk to many people who hated high school. I loved it!

Getting Married

The summer between my junior and senior year of high school I was dating a guy who was in college. We kinda, sorta, almost had sex. One of my friends got pregnant and came to talk to my mother about it. I realized I was later on my period than she was. I could not go to the doctor to find out for sure. That would be admitting I wasn't a good girl!

Two days later, my boyfriend and I went to Mexico and got married. I was scared to death. A guide on the street took us and our money out into the middle of what seemed like nowhere. I could see us disappearing forever. Finally, in a small courthouse about sixty miles from the border, I said, "I do", I think. It was in Spanish so I am not for sure, however, I did have a valid marriage license. My mother and husband altered our marriage license, changing the Julio to Junio. That way people would never know I was pregnant when I got married. This was a well-planned, carefully executed lie. My Dad didn't know the truth for 26 years. He would tell people I had the longest pregnancy – six and a half years.

My husband's parents wanted three hundred wedding announcements sent out to their friends and business associates. They wanted it to have my hometown printed on them rather than Mexico. So now, the date and the place were fabricated. This was a secret that would go to the grave with me. Two weeks later, I started my period.

My College Years

A month later, I moved a hundred miles away to the large university town where my new husband was a student. I went to night school to finish my senior year. My husband went to class, worked half-days and studied in the evenings. We only had one car. We were living in a small apartment where everyone else was really old, at *least* 20 years old. We had very, very little money. I was home alone all day. I was so miserable. I went from having all of my friends around to having no one around. I returned to my two best friends, food and reading.

I got a job to relieve the boredom and help with the bills. The first week on the assignment, an older man asked me to go for coffee. I was shocked! I was married. I knew how to flirt when I was single but I was married now. I gained ten pounds the first month. The more weight I gained, the less male-attention was a problem. However, clothes were. I had lots of clothes that mother had made me when I lived at home. We had no money for new ones, besides why buy clothes when I was going to lose weight?

I think it was harder to lose weight and regain it because I knew what life was like not being fat. I had lived the Ugly Duckling story and now I had gone back to being the ugly duck again. I knew a normal person was in there.

I finished high school in three months and started at the university in January. There were 550 students in my math class. My entire high school enrollment was 375 for all four grades! I went home to visit my high school friends one week. They were talking about "who was talking to who in the halls at school"; I was worried about the cost of tuna fish. I felt very, very old.

I heard smoking kept you from eating. I started and it worked. I felt sick and wasn't hungry. I eventually learned the best time for a cigarette was after a huge meal. One more addiction. In the beginning, I didn't smoke in front of my husband for several reasons. I knew it would prevent me from becoming a really heavy smoker. I knew at an early age that I have an addictive personality. (Thank God, that knowledge kept me from trying drugs or I might be living on the streets by now.) Smoking was also a very good rebellion. No one wanted me to smoke. Not my parents, husband, in-laws, society, my doctors. So, whenever I got mad, I would smoke. Sometimes, two cigarettes.

The next summer I went on my own invented "hamburger and peach diet". I would have a hamburger for lunch and a peach for dinner. That was around 500 calories. I lost 20 pounds in about a month. The antibiotics and medical bill shot our budget. Someone said I would get sick on that diet. They were right. Honestly, I do remember thinking, "When people walk up to look at me in my casket, at least I will be thin!"

My best friend was a 78 years old spinster and I was 18. At least once a week, she would bring over food from a local deli. They made the very worst banana pudding I have ever tasted! It was so bad, it took me two days to eat it. I could only eat a few bites at a time and put it back in the refrigerator for a few more hours.

My husband graduated from the university and we moved to his hometown. He started working with his father at a family- owned business. I started commuting to a woman's university thirty miles from home. I knew where every vending machine was in every building. There was an ice cream shop beside the parking lot with great strawberry cheesecake ice cream. There was a fast food restaurant on the corner of the highway with wonderful, cheap tacos and fries. I ate. I dieted. I ate. I dieted. I ate.

I made no friends at either university. I have no yearbooks, no photographs of me. It is like I only existed during those years. I remember no one, but I remember the chili-covered burritos at the student union building.

I went shopping at an outlet store to try to find something to wear. I hated going up sizes so I would look for the loosest outfit. I went to the dressing room and pulled the dress over my head and I got stuck in it. It wouldn't come on or go off. I panicked which caused me to sweat and become more stuck. I'll never forget that moment.

I, of course, was an eventful dieter. I had to go on a diet for every event in my life. One May, my sister-in-law announced her wedding, that would take place in September, and I was one of the bridesmaids. The dresses were fitted and my mother-in-law wanted me to get mine made early. This was impossible because I had no idea what size I would be then. I wanted to lose 25 pounds before the wedding. If I got the dress made before I lost weight, it wouldn't fit. If I lost weight and got the dress made too soon, what if I gained it back before the big night? I felt scared and panicky. Besides, how do you explain that kind of dilemma to normal people?

I would yo-yo. I weighed 140 and I was never going to weigh more than that! I lost down to 135. I weighed 150 and I was really never going to weigh more that that! I lost down to 135. I weighed 160 and I was really never, ever going to weigh more than that! I lost down to 135. I weighed 167 and I was really, really never ever going to weigh more than that!

I never weighed except in the morning. If I crept up on the scale and pointed it to the northeast, I weighed less. The Scale God would give me my daily judgment. "Thou art a good person because your weight is down or Thou art a horrible person because you have gained." I never quite understood how the same number on the scale felt so good on the way down and so horrible on the way back up.

Teaching School

I started teaching kindergarten the first year it was required in our state. I requested the low-income, predominately minority school. I had a classroom of 22 boys and 12 girls. I had two tables and 20 chairs and no equipment when school began. I will never forget that first day of school. I looked at that sea of faces and squirming, warm little bodies and I thought, "Oh, my God, they didn't teach me how to do this!" I knew theory and textbooks – not how to get 34 kids through the lunch line, open milk cartons, eat, clean up our places and get out of the lunchroom in 20 minutes. If we were late, the entire school was late.

Once I was on a famous clinic diet that was making the rounds. There were very specific foods you ate at each meal; Saturday was all the fruit you could eat. Well, Tuesday's lunch was two boiled eggs and a cup of spinach; cold as there were no microwave ovens back then. I tried to swallow them without really chewing, just to get them down. My class was standing in line as we were leaving the lunchroom and one little girl had thrown up her lunch on her fake fur coat. I ate those wonderful fresh sugar cookies in the teacher's lounge that afternoon. I never made it to the fruit on Saturday. After it got fuzzy in the refrigerator several weeks later, I threw it out.

Occasionally, I would buy two boxes of chocolate covered peanuts. I would hide one in the utility room, then come in the living room and share the other box with my husband. Later, when he was asleep, I had my own box all to myself. I would sometimes go in the bathroom and lock the door and eat. No one else was even home at the time.

I lost weight that next summer. Generally, when I hit 135 I would reward myself with some new clothes, several really cute tight outfits. Some had tags still on them because I would regain the weight so soon. I usually maintained my weight loss as long as it took me to walk from my bathroom scales to the kitchen. They would hang in my closet for years because on Monday, I was going on a diet and lose the weight. I wore the same couple of pair of stretch pants and baggy blouses, day in and a day out. I never wanted to waste money on fat clothes because I was going on my diet tomorrow and it would be wasting money. My friends wore hip-huggers and halter-tops. I wore muu-muu dresses that covered everything and touched nothing. I felt embarrassed, ashamed, old and ugly, even though people said I had such a pretty face. I was twenty-three.

I continued going to graduate school while I taught and also during the summers. Finally, all I needed to complete my Master's Degree in Early Childhood Education was my professional paper. The same week I started the semester, I learned my mother was dying and was told she had only six months to a year to live. My heart sank every time the telephone rang. I could not handle the stress of my paper and Momma dying.

My mother found a recommendation for one of the best gynecologists in Dallas because even though cervical cancer isn't hereditary, the tendency does run in families. I had two months before my first appointment so I went on a diet and lost 12 pounds. I didn't want him to yell at me about my weight. That backfired on me. When I regained that weight, just getting back to where I had started, it looked like a weight gain on my chart. Oh, well.

First Pregnancy - Myka

My mother wanted a grandbaby and my husband wanted a child. We had been married six years and everyone was ready but me. I was enjoying teaching. I looked at my life. I had a degree, a wedding ring, a brand new house – everything a little girl dreams about, except a baby. I thought that was the only thing I had to look forward to in the future. Babies were such a big responsibility for life! Momma and my husband talked and talked and "guilted" me into getting pregnant. It is a decision I have never regretted.

I did well on my weight when I was pregnant. I always did because I knew I would be weighed regularly. Remember, I don't like to be yelled at about my weight. I gained about 20 pounds and weighed less on my first checkup than pre-pregnancy.

Momma came over from my parent's home forty-five miles away to help me celebrate my 24th birthday; it was two weeks past my due date. I went into labor and she helped me count the contractions. I have always thought that was a miracle that I could share that with her. She went to get my dad as we went to the hospital.

The next morning my daughter, Myka, was born. Mother was really sick and passing big clots of blood, but she wouldn't go to her hospital because she was afraid she would never be able to hold her only grandbaby. I came home three days later. Mother and Dad spent the night and held Myka. Mother went to the hospital the next day.

Mother's Death

Mother was in and out of the hospital many times that winter. We thought she would have to spend her last Christmas in it. Momma loved Christmas and made it such a big production for the entire family. She got out on Christmas Eve and we spent it at the Ranch with my aunts, uncles, and cousins. Another miracle was that she had very little pain for two days and seemed much like her funny, joking self. The leaving was so sad that year because we all knew it would be her last Christmas and she was saying her last goodbyes to many family members.

Momma spent nearly the last two months of her life in the hospital. I was visiting her at the big Dallas hospital as often as possible. I had a house, a five-month-old child, husband and a dying mother. She was in so much pain. She smelled of death. The holes cut in her body wouldn't heal.

One day, she said, "If I took all of my pain medication at once, it would be over. I'm afraid God wouldn't forgive me, but He would forgive you for killing me." Many days as I watched her fall into a fitful sleep, I would think, 'I could just put the pillow over her face and all of her suffering would be over'. I would snap out of those thoughts with utter horror. How could I even imagine killing this woman I loved so much? She was only 45. They would find a cure next week. They would do something to save her life. Still, the thought plagues me. I wanted her pain to stop.

We talked about her funeral and where she wanted her things to go. We talked about death, her death. We read books. We made amends to each other for anything we had done or said to harm the other. We laughed. We cried. We hugged and held each other as we waited for death to take her.

A steamy day in June, she asked me for a favor. "Anything you want, Momma!" She said, "Please go on a diet and lose weight before my funeral. All your old friends from high school are going to come and I don't want them to see you as fat as you are."

I had lost 17 pounds and bought a cute new long skirt to wear to a party on Friday. I brought it to model for her. (I never did get to wear it.) Mother had finally fallen off to sleep about the time I was to leave the hospital in order to avoid rush hour traffic. Her doctor said there was some improvement and she could possibly go home for the weekend. I kissed her forehead and told her I loved her. I remember walking down that long hallway towards the elevator still feeling that kiss on my lips.

The next morning about 5:30 AM, my father called to say mother was dead. I wore a maternity dress that had a belt with it to her funeral. I sat in the funeral home, ashamed that I was still too fat and thinking my mother wanted me thinner. I was so grateful one of my previous boyfriends was on vacation and unable to come because he would have seen me fat but his parents were there.

We went back to Grannie's and there was so much food people had brought in. I didn't eat for a while and then I started with the homemade chocolate meringue pies. I came home, closed the blinds, didn't answer the phone and ate and ate and ate. As long as people didn't say they were sorry to hear about Momma, I could hold in the tears in public. I mainly cried when I was embarrassed and crying embarrassed me! So it was easier to eat and read and hide and isolate.

One night, a few weeks after Mother had died, I was crying late at night. Myka was usually sleeping through the night, but she woke up crying. As I rocked her back to sleep, I thought, 'If my children can love me as much as I loved my mother, I will be okay.'

Most of my life consisted of staying up late after my husband went to bed. I was smoking, reading romance novels and bingeing, getting up in the morning, lying on the couch, reading, eating, watching television, snacking, eating dinner, and after he went to bed, smoking, reading romance novels and bingeing again and again and again. When I would go to bed, my thoughts would flood my mind. "You forgot to mail off the payment for the book club. You need to mail out those thank you cards. You have got to write that paper to finish your Master's Degree."

I would wake up exhausted and think, "Oh, shit, it is another day." I had nothing to look forward to doing. I would check out the cookie can. I would eat, drink 6 quart bottles of diet drink, smoke, read, worry, cry, eat, read, and smoke. Tell myself what I should be doing. Ignore what I should be doing. Feel guilty. Eat. Over and over and over again.

Reunion Time

My husband's ten-year high school reunion was coming up in June. I knew he would insist on going and my going with him. I couldn't embarrass him, being as fat as I was; his old girlfriends would be there.

I went on a low-carb diet a neighbor had given me. Before she moved to our town, she had been to some meetings of a Twelve-Step recovery program for compulsive overeaters. It was the organization's recommended food plan. We decided to go on it together. She quit after four days. I was really desperate so I stayed on it for 5 weeks and lost 25 pounds. I felt pretty good about it but wanted to lose more.

Then, my aunt told me **THE SECRET**. I was so pissed no one had told me before now. She said to stay on my diet during the week and allow myself to eat a meal on Saturday and Sunday of anything I wanted including dessert. That was how she maintained her weight. It was so simple, why didn't I think of it? What a wonderful new plan!

The next Monday, someone asked me to play bridge in the ladies' bridge club. There were always great desserts. I decided to go back on my "diet" on Tuesday instead. Then, on Tuesday, I would remember, "Thou shalt not start a diet on any day except Monday or New Year's Day." I would then have to eat all my "Last Suppers" until the next Monday. I would go to all my favorite places to eat the one last time before the diet started. Then, on Monday, another friend would ask me to play bridge and it started all over again. It was as if I "came to" in November. I stepped on the scale and I had gained all of the weight I'd lost, plus interest.

Second Pregnancy -Mekala

This next spring I got pregnant again. I had continued to avoid writing my professional paper to finish my Master's Degree but many nights I thought about it. I hated it when people asked if I had written it yet. There is a five-year time limit on completing a Master's and I was quickly approaching the deadline. There is a quote, "Procrastination and masturbation are alike in that it feels good at first, but you end up screwing yourself."

I forced myself to write it and it took me all of two weeks. I walked out of my meeting with my committee where I defended it; it took 15 minutes. As I walked down that hallway, I thought, "I can not believe you spent five years worrying, dreading, and obsessing about that paper and it only took two weeks to do it."

During my pregnancy, I craved green tomato relish but it isn't something I felt like eating by itself. So, I cooked two sourdough rolls for 10 minutes. That was so good I cooked two more for 10 more minutes. That was so very good I cooked two more for another 10 minutes. I ended up eating 10 rolls with butter. I would have never considered cooking all 10 of them because I was only going to eat 2. That was the longest binge I can recall.

Again, I lost 10 pounds by the time I brought Mekala home from the hospital. Remember, I don't like doctors yelling at me? I tried my size 16 jeans with a 34-inch waist. They were about 8 inches from meeting in the front. I wore one pair of blue stretch pants and 2 blouses and one dress any time I was in public. My goal of the day was to not stay in my gown all day long. I had 3 muu-muus and I tried to not wear the same one for two days in a row.

First Time at Twelve Step Programs

A friend called me and told me she was going to a twelve-step recovery program for compulsive overeaters. I decided to give it a try since I had lost 25 pounds on their food plan two years earlier, getting ready for my husband's reunion. I had to find an overweight friend to go with me because I couldn't go anywhere by myself. I knew that night, these people had lived the same hell with food I had.

I'll never forget what my friend said to me on the way home from the meeting. "I never knew your weight bothered you." I had been with this woman at least 4 times a week for 10 years and she didn't know my weight bothered me! I thought about it constantly.

I read somewhere many years ago about a personality disorder. It described a person who people, after five minutes, felt they knew everything about him/her. The person was very talkative, telling about their friends, vacations, past experiences, etc. The problem was that they knew as much in five minutes as they did in five years because he/she only told them exactly what he/she wanted them to know. My friend knew so much about my "life" but nothing about my feelings.

At the meeting, I bought all of the literature they had available which I think was a few pamphlets and the Alcoholics Anonymous[1] (Big Book) and The Twelve Steps and Twelve Traditions of Alcoholics Anonymous.[2] (12 and 12) I had hope. The next week I had to find a different overweight friend to go with me since I still couldn't go alone. The third week I found another person to go with me. I still couldn't go alone. The food plan was very restrictive. I was hungry, my baby was crying, I wanted to climb the walls. (By the way, that and jumping to conclusions were my favorite exercises.)

I read the literature and I identified. Really, I identified all the *other* people I knew whose life could be improved by following this simple program.

I couldn't be on that food plan and nurse my daughter. I didn't produce enough milk and she would cry. I would eat cookies and, miraculously, I would produce more. I always knew cookies and milk went together. I did not go back the fourth week.

Serious Disease Time

I really loved bundt cakes. I could cut a big piece and then squeeze it together so it looked like only a small piece was gone. I would bake a cake or pie then, it called my name, "Tonna, I'm waiting in the kitchen for you. Just one piece." I would white knuckle it for a few days, really wanting to eat it all, then and there. Finally, thank goodness, it would finally be gone. A week later, my husband would ask me if there was any of that cake left. I wanted to hit him! He had no idea how much I had fought with myself over that stupid cake.

A friend brought me some banana-nut bread when I came home from the hospital with Mekala. It came from the donut shop and it was wonderful. I would buy a loaf and sliver it to death. Every time I went through the room, I would eat a piece. My husband didn't really like it much but sometimes, he would ask for a piece. Silently, I resented having to share. Finally, one loaf wasn't enough to last me for a day and I started to buy two a day and eat them both.

I think all of my addictions may boil down to being addicted to "next". The first bite was good and I noticed how wonderful the last bite was, but I couldn't remember all the in-between bites. After I stopped eating, I would mentally go, "NEXT" and get another bowl of ice cream or some chips. So, it was the next diet drink, the next alcoholic drink, the next cigarette, the next romance novel, the next cookie, the next donut, the next vacation, on and on and on.

Many times I needed to go to the grocery store to buy milk for my children; life was simpler when the kids had milk for cereal in the mornings. I could not find the motivation to get dressed and go; however, if I wanted some dip and a bag of chips, I would make up an excuse and go in the middle of the night. I could always say I needed some feminine products. Isn't it amazing the lengths I would go to get what I wanted but not what I needed?

One day I had some place nice I needed to go. I sat in my closet floor surrounded by many sizes of clothes, crying because nothing fit. Talk about feeling sad, hopeless, scared and discouraged. I was 27 and I felt my life was over.

My OB/Gyn told me the best time to lose weight was while breast-feeding. I gained 17 pounds in six months. I had a check-up scheduled so I decided I had to lose it. I went on the 500 of my usual "500 or 5000 calorie a day diet". I could not stay on my diet until 10 AM before I would start emptying out the cookie can. I was really scared because, before, I could always stop.

My MD said nothing about my weight at my appointment. I sat in the parking garage, relieved about it. Then, I thought 'he knows it is of no use. I will always be fat, so why bother talking to me about it?'

I decided to live my life as a fat person. I would wear sleeveless clothes. I would not deprive my children of experiences because of my weight. I wore a bright yellow cover-up to the swimming pool where Mekala was taking a water-babies class. One of my husband's old classmates was there in a bikini and I felt like Big Bird. During class, I sunk down in the water where only my head stuck out, a difficult task in 3-foot water.

Our next-door neighbors invited another couple and us over to play cards. The wife served a really delicious dessert. She wasn't having any and someone remarked on it. She said, "My husband doesn't want a fat wife." I knew neither did mine. I almost cried I was so embarrassed. I know she didn't mean to say something that would hurt me, but I was publicly humiliated.

One night I noticed a prong on my wedding ring set was loose. I tried to take the ring off. I was so fat I couldn't get it over my knuckles. I tried everything I could think of, ice water, soap, shortening, wrapping thread around my finger, to no avail. I woke up my husband and he said, "Don't worry about it, come to bed." My finger was swelling and throbbing by this time. I remembered a fireman telling me that he sometimes had to cut off rings. I called the fire station. The dispatcher said, "Yes, we do. We'll send out an ambulance." My in-laws lived three doors down from us. I could imagine what they and all the neighbors would think with sirens and flashing lights at 2 AM.

I told them I would come there instead. I wanted to wake my husband and have him take me, but I had two sleeping children. I went alone. Embarrassed that in 10 years I had gained that much weight, I drove to the fire station. I joked with the fireman who cut it off. "Oh, it is gold all the way through, so he didn't buy it at the convenience store after all." He commented to the other one, "She sure is feeling good tonight." I wondered if they thought I had been drinking. I have had few nights where I felt so humiliated and embarrassed.

The next morning my husband asked me why my finger swelled up so much. I said, "I guess a spider bit me on it." What, admit I had just got too fat? I couldn't get the jeweler to repair my rings because I didn't want to make my rings larger because I was going on a diet, on Monday.

I was desperate. I decided I would fast. I woke up at 9:00 full of determination. My husband came home for lunch. I told him I wish we'd gone to eat fast-food fried fish one last time. He said, "Why don't we go tonight?" Great, here I already had 3 long hours of fasting. I couldn't stop thinking about that fish and chips. At three o'clock, I called him and told him we would make the 40-mile round trip to eat it.

I was starving and it would be at least 3-4 hours before we could eat. I made chicken salad and ate all of it and a whole sleeve of crackers. No one else liked it and I didn't need leftovers tomorrow when I started my fast again. I was still so stuffed when we went to eat. However, I ate all of my order and what my daughter didn't eat of hers because it might be my "Last Supper" for a long, long time. I thought I would explode on the drive home. I don't remember what happened the next day, but I didn't fast. Probably had to wait until the next Monday.

Next, I went on the starvation soup diet. It was a recipe that I made in my five-gallon spaghetti pot. It had a whole head of cabbage, 6 tomatoes, an entire bunch of celery, 2 onions and it could be lightly sprinkled with Parmesan cheese. The theory was that it took more calories to digest it than the soup contained. The greatest words ever to a compulsive overeater, "You can eat all you want". I was supposed to eat a bowl about every two hours but I think my dirty dishwater probably had more flavor than it did.

I ate three bowls the first day and poured the rest out a week later when the refrigerator began to stink. I knew it was too good to be true.

Trying One More Time

In October of 1979, I went back to that twelve-step program. I was desperate. **My** ten-year high school reunion was coming up and I could not go fat and I wanted to see my friends that I had avoided as much as possible for all these years. I knew by this time, no matter what the magazines at the grocery store checkout lines said, I could not lose 50 pounds in 3 weeks.

I came home from the meeting and I hugged my husband because I could not stand the intimacy of looking at him. I told him I had to do this recovery deal for the rest of my life because I did not want to go on living, if I had to live like this. My recovery had begun. If you are interested in recovering, you may turn this book over and read about my recovery. You will also find 500 practical things you can do to help you recover. There is no magic, but I do believe in miracles. I believe I am one.

[1] Alcoholics Anonymous, ©1939, 1955, 1976, 2001, Alcoholics
        Anonymous World Services, Inc.
[2] The Twelve Steps and Twelve Traditions of Alcoholics Anonymous
        ©1953, Alcoholics Anonymous World Services, Inc.

My Story – The Recovery is located in 500 Solutions

Side B

Chapter One

Chapter Three

500 Excuses

We are all tired of our excuses and those of others. My friend always says, "Excuses are like assholes, everybody has one." Here is a list of 500 excuses you may use. I used many of them on a regular basis before I got into recovery 26 years ago. You can get some new ideas. Be creative.

You may have a binge buddy with whom you can share these. When you become familiar enough with them, you can say, "I am 6, 29, 299 and 436 today" Your buddy will be able to respond, "I am 43, 92, 377, and 412." It can be your own language.

You can write random numbers on each day of your calendar. Then, look up that number on the list and you can only use that excuse and no other one for the next 24 hours. You may want to make a flip chart with a new one for the week. You can make a screensaver with your numbers or excuses to remind you each day.

Some of the excuses are valid, logical, and some are goofy. I do not intend to offend anyone. I am not picking on anyone or making fun of people. I am not minimizing or discounting your feelings or beliefs.

Most of the overweight women and men I have counseled have reported some sexual trauma. There are many, many studies that link sexual abuse to overeating. If you are interested, please look it up at the library or on the Internet.

If you are dissatisfied with any of the excuses or want a new one, just contact me at the following email address: Tonna@overeating500solutions.com and I will send a different one. I have not included them all. I just needed a place to stop.

I double-spaced them so you can edit or adapt the ones I have listed. You may want to write whatever feelings you experience when you read them.

Here are my 500 Excuses:

1. I am a big eater.

2. I was made to clean my plate.

3. I am a Southerner and love chicken-fried steak and gravy.

4. I never got to eat out as a child.

5. I ate fast food all the time as a child because my mother never cooked.

6. I have a glandular problem.

7. I have big bones.

8. I have an under-active thyroid.

9. I never lost my baby fat.

10. I am Mexican and mother always made fresh tortillas every meal.

11. I am using my weight to avoid being sexual.

12. I am fat to punish my husband.

13. My mother always tried to make me lose weight.

14. My mother is a great cook.

15. My family showed love with food.

16. I never have time to cook food that's healthy.

17. I am lonely and food is my friend.

18. I really don't eat much.

19. I don't have time to exercise.

20. I hate vegetables.

21. I was always a spoiled child.

22. I am Catholic.

23. My parents didn't love me enough.

24. I wasn't wanted.

25. I was sexually abused.

26. I have slow metabolism.

27. I am afraid of being attractive.

28. I get to blame my lack of success on my weight.

29. I get to avoid people.

30. I am African-American.

31. Eating is my only social outlet.

32. My grandmother was such a good cook.

33. I don't like to sweat.

34. I am a chocoholic.

35. I love bread.

36. I am too short.

37. I would go to bed without enough to eat as a child.

38. I am afraid of being hungry.

39. I never lost weight after I had my babies.

40. It is too cold to exercise.

41. I ate for two when I was pregnant.

42. I ate with my wife when she was pregnant.

43. I feel more powerful when I am fat.

44. It is a power struggle with my husband.

45. No one will ever want to be with me, so why not?

46. I am a loser.

47. I really ate big as a football player and just continued to eat that way.

48. I do hard physical labor and I need that much food.

49. I am too lazy to cook.

50. All the women in my family are large.

51. I just have a big butt.

52. I have heavy thighs and it runs in my family.

53. I can't stop drinking soft drinks.

54. I graze all day.

55. I grab food on the run.

56. I never can get a chance to sit down to eat.

57. Eating is safe sex.

58. Eating calms me down.

59. I always have a snack in the afternoon.

60. I have to get up in the night and snack.

61. I can't go to bed without a full tummy.

62. I love cereal.

63. I can't seem to be able to push away from the table.

64. I am a great cook.

65. I love watching the food television shows.

66. I live near a bakery.

67. I adore doughnuts.

68. I had a candy store next to my school.

69. I have to have a soft drink in the morning to get started.

70. My mother was obsessed with her weight.

71. My mother was obsessed with my weight.

72. My husband likes fat women.

73. I am Brazilian.

74. My wife likes big men.

75. I am vertically challenged.

76. It is a power struggle with my wife.

77. It is a beer gut.

78. Christians can't get together without desserts.

79. My Jewish mother feeds me all the time.

80. It would hurt my friend's feeling if I don't eat what they cook for me.

81. I have to have ice cream every night.

82. I am Portuguese.

83. Food soothes my nerves.

84. I work in a restaurant.

85. I eat when I get nervous.

86. My office is always having big spreads.

87. I eat out with co-workers at lunch.

88. There is always a birthday celebration at work.

89. My co-workers have a full candy jar at all times.

90. I am Russian.

91. I am British and we ate big breakfasts.

92. My parents owned a store and I could have all the food I wanted.

93. I am not going to be deprived.

94. My food is so monitored that I sneak food.

95. I hide food from others.

96. I have to eat in private because I am ashamed of my eating.

97. I am Italian, need I say more.

98. Nobody is going to tell me what I can and cannot eat.

99. Food is my fun.

100. My husband and I entertain all the time.

101. I am a great hostess.

102. I have to take clients out to eat nearly every day.

103. I am Canadian.

104. I retain water.

105. I don't have time to cook vegetables.

106. I love fried foods.

107. I am Christian.

108. My mother always cooked with bacon grease.

109. I lived on a farm and had biscuits and gravy every morning.

110. I am French and you know what kind of pastries we have.

111. We ate potatoes every day.

112. I had to steal food as a child.

113. I am a Native American.

114. I spent all my money on food as a child.

115. My father would make comments about my body.

116. My siblings called me "fatty".

117. I am Jewish.

118. It is too hot to exercise.

119. I am Irish.

120. I love pasta.

121. I have to have my daily candy bars.

122. I am afraid to be thin.

123. My mother would not allow us to eat sugar.

124. I eat when I am anxious.

125. I sit in front of the computer all the time.

126. There is no safe place to walk in my neighborhood.

127. I am Indian.

128. I cannot afford low-calorie food.

129. I drink a six-pack of sodas a day.

130. My knees are too bad to exercise.

131. I am Muslim.

132. I love to try new ethnic foods.

133. My boss drives me crazy.

134. I can only eat one meal a day.

135. I cannot eat breakfast because it makes my stomach hurt.

136. I am compulsive about nuts.

137. I have no friends.

138. I was fat as a child.

139. I was sick as a child and everyone kept feeding me.

140. I was too skinny as a child.

141. I got tired of puking up my food to be thin.

142. I refuse to diet ever again.

143. My husband gets too jealous when I lose weight.

144. I am Spanish.

145. I am a Northerner.

146. No one likes me.

147. I am hard to get along with and food is my only friend.

148. I am just not in the mood to diet.

149. I am Hawaiian.

150. I grew up on grits.

151. I am Norwegian.

152. I use food to stuff down my anger.

153. I eat so I don't feel.

154. I eat when I need to be comforted.

155. I love Chinese food.

156. Food is the one constant in my life.

157. I eat when I am happy.

158. I eat when I am sad.

159. I eat when I am frustrated.

160. I eat when I am mad.

161. I eat when I am tired.

162. I need a salt/sugar fix like popcorn and a sweet soft drink.

163. Food gives me energy.

164. No one is going to mess with "MY" food.

165. I keep a hidden food stash.

166. I sneak food.

167. I have to get in the mood to lose weight.

168. I am Caribbean.

169. I am a food inspector.

170. I make homemade bread with my grandmother's sourdough starter every two days.

171. I work in a bakery.

172. All my friends are overweight.

173. I cannot stay on a diet.

174. I am Japanese.

175. My wife and I are binge buddies.

176. I know I won't be tempted to cheat on my spouse if I am overweight.

177. I can blame everything on my "weight".

178. I have an excuse for everything.

179. My friends wouldn't like me if I was dieting.

180. I am too irritable when I get hungry.

181. I am Chinese.

182. I do not like much protein, only starches.

183. I hate all green vegetables.

184. I am rebellious.

185. Why should I be thin?

186. Who says I should look like all those skinny models?

60

187. I am Thai.

188. Thin people are too stuck on themselves.

189. I should not have to lose weight to get a date.

190. I am Cambodian.

191. Men are jerks for not liking my weight.

192. If people do not like how I look, they can stop looking.

193. Fresh fruits and vegetables spoil too quickly.

194. I am addicted to sugar.

195. It is fault of the capitalist pig businesses.

196. I love snack foods.

197. I do not eat at regular meal times.

198. Why does the media get to determine what is beautiful?

199. I do not have time to go to any recovery meetings.

200. Sometimes I eat all the food and have to make more so my family won't know.

201. I am painfully shy.

202. I get to pretend that I am a "jolly" fat person.

203. I get to hide behind my fat.

204. I am Columbian.

205. I have to have lots of carbs to get energy.

206. I am Vietnamese.

207. I graze.

208. I am on welfare and food stamps and the cheap food is fattening.

209. I never eat during the day.

210. Food is my reward.

211. I am German.

212. I eat too late at night.

213. I am bombarded with food all day.

214. I work at night and eating keeps me awake.

215. You would be fat too, if you had *my* family.

216. I crave Mexican food.

217. I am never home.

218. I am home all day with my children.

219. I cannot afford to join a gym.

220. I have no self-discipline.

221. I am just like an alcoholic, except my drug of choice is food!

222. I don't know about nutrition.

223. I buy food in bulk because it is so much cheaper.

224. What would Thanksgiving be without bingeing?

225. I am no dietitian.

226. I show love with food.

227. I put love in my food when I cook.

228. My mother gave me food to reward me.

229. My father would send me to bed without any food as punishment.

230. I was punished for not cleaning my plate.

231. Women like big, strong men.

232. I am afraid of liposuction.

233. I am going go get my stomach stapled when I get time.

234. I retain water.

235. My husband is a gourmet cook.

236. I hate cooking.

237. I read recipe books for fun.

238. I have tried dieting before and it did not work.

239. I have gone to so many weight loss programs and they do not work.

240. My wife sabotages my food plan.

241. I live in New York City - do I need to say more?

242. I love Italian food!

243. I clean my children's plates.

244. I am the garbage disposal when I clean up the kitchen.

245. It is the food industry's fault.

246. I can eat a whole large pizza by myself.

247. People would have higher expectations of me.

248. My Dad fed me so I would be a big football player.

249. I am Iraqi.

250. Exercise takes too much time.

251. Every other commercial on television is about some junk food.

252. We were poor when I was growing up.

253. I don't like to waste food.

254. I am not really all that fat.

255. I am Nigerian.

256. I can't stop thinking about food.

257. I have to eat the Valentine candy my sweetheart buys me.

258. I am a compulsive overeater.

259. I have no idea how to stop it.

260. I have no self-esteem.

261. My parents loved me too much.

262. I am Iranian.

263. I love rich sauces.

264. I am a gourmet cook.

265. I have no idea how to eat healthy.

266. My parents were wealthy and we ate at wonderful restaurants.

267. I just enjoy eating.

268. You can't celebrate without food!

269. Life wouldn't be worth living if I couldn't eat.

270. I love movies and I have to have popcorn and soft drinks.

271. Whenever I date, we always go out to eat.

272. My friends expect me to eat with them.

273. I've always been fat.

274. It is just in my genes.

275. I would have to give up my identity to be thin.

276. I don't know if I could trust the opposite sex if I were attractive.

277. You can't expect me not to eat all those Christmas goodies.

278. I am from California and I love Sourdough bread from San Francisco with lots of real butter!

279. I love Thai food with all the peanut sauces.

280. I like real food and not all that fat-free crap.

281. I associate certain food with special times.

282. God gave us all these foods to enjoy.

283. The economy would collapse if I stopped eating!

284. I am Scottish.

285. It is the government's fault.

286. Everything is bigger in Texas.

287. I am Cajun and can we cook!

288. I live on fries and hamburgers.

289. You can't diet when you travel as much as I do.

290. I love malts and shakes.

291. I don't like seafood.

292. I am Lebanese.

293. I bake cakes all the time.

294. I am Swedish.

295. I never met a carb I didn't like.

296. I'll never go hungry again.

297. I hate skinny girls.

298. My comfort foods bring me back a sense of safety.

299. My Dad would take me to get ice cream when I was a child and I loved those times.

300. I am a Saudi Arabian.

301. Kids made fun of me at school.

302. I can't afford a whole new wardrobe.

303. I crave food all the time.

304. I think my friends would resent me if I lost weight.

305. I don't know if I could trust me if I was thin.

306. I know I couldn't keep it off, even if I lost it.

307. I am from the Midwest.

308. I've lost and gained it back so many times so what's the use?

309. It is a chicken way of killing myself.

310. I have given up.

311. I just have cellulite.

312. I am Panamanian.

313. I go on cruises every year and I eat all day long.

314. I travel with my job so I can't eat right.

315. The experts change their minds about every 5 years so who knows what is right.

316. I am healthy at this weight.

317. My whole family is overweight.

318. I have always been the "fat one" in the family.

319. I am Hungarian.

320. I don't really care what I am eating as long as it is food.

321. I am afraid I will never get enough.

322. I never get full.

323. I don't know what healthy serving sizes are.

324. A whole package is my idea of a serving.

325. It is my father's fault.

326. I have an empty hole in my soul.

327. Get off my back!

328. I can eat myself to death and my family won't know, I really killed myself.

329. I am Korean.

330. I can't stop when I am full.

331. I eat past the stuffed point regularly.

332. I have no self-discipline.

333. I am Jamaican.

334. I start a diet every Monday morning and it never works.

335. I am so tired of people talking about my size!

336. Why should I have to lose weight to please you?

337. I am Peruvian.

338. Food is entertainment.

339. I came from a big family and we are always having family get-togethers.

340. My mother thinks if I am not fat, I will be sick.

341. I am an agnostic.

342. I get frustrated with diet food.

343. I can't afford to go to diet doctors.

344. I am Polynesian.

345. I don't see the point of working so hard to lose weight.

346. Why should I?

347. I know it is going to take a commitment and I am not ready yet.

348. I have gone so far that there isn't any hope for me.

349. No one understands me.

350. I grew up during the depression.

351. I am depressed.

352. My medication makes me fat.

353. I am too old to lose weight.

354. I am just fat and happy.

355. Just leave me alone!

356. I am digging my grave with a fork.

357. I am Cuban.

358. If I didn't have to work, I would be fine.

359. The nuns made us eat at school.

360. I came home to an empty house after school and the pantry had such goodies.

361. I am Lutheran.

362. My mother always had treats for me when I came home from school.

363. My grandmother would bake me all of my favorites.

364. If I had a job, I wouldn't eat all day.

365. When I went to the doctor and got a shot, I got a sucker.

366. I always had money for the ice cream truck.

367. I would steal money from my parents to buy candy.

368. I make up lies to leave the house so I can get my food.

369. My abuser would buy me food to keep me quiet about the abuse.

370. My mother was a horrible cook.

371. I lived in filth as a child.

372. I am Polish.

373. I had to take my lunch to school every day.

374. I could never please my parents.

375. I had to eat school food.

376. I was on free lunches at school and I was embarrassed.

377. My mother made fun of my body.

378. I ate to cover up my body.

379. I was scared of men's attention, in fact, I still am.

380. I would have to be more responsible for myself.

381. I have too much responsibility.

382. If I can't diet perfectly, why try?

383. I was horrible in gym class and I have a phobia of exercise.

384. I can't go to aerobics because I have nothing I could wear.

385. If I didn't have to go to social events, I could diet.

386. If I wasn't married, I could be thin.

387. I just love food!

388. If I didn't live alone, I could be a normal eater.

389. In Florida, I play cards and we snack all day.

390. I am Greek.

391. I am scared of not having enough.

392. My siblings would threaten to tell about my eating.

393. At least the whole package was fat-free.

394. I need something in the afternoon to give me energy.

395. I always had to share my goodies with my brother.

396. I steal my kids Halloween candy and have to go buy them more.

397. I am a Jehovah's Witness.

398. I have to hide my candy wrappers.

399. I have to go to different fast food places because I am embarrassed to eat so much.

400. I get clothes with pockets so I can hide food.

401. I have an excuse for not being sexual.

402. I am Taiwanese.

403. I don't have to compete.

404. I have a reason to hate myself.

405. When I was sick, my mother would make me special foods.

406. I was forced to eat foods I hated.

407. When I got good grades, my parents rewarded me with food!

408. I love romantic dinners.

409. I am a Mormon.

410. Look at Buddha; he was spiritual and fat.

411. People would laugh at me in exercise class.

412. People are so rude to me about my weight.

413. My family is in denial about my unhealthy weight.

414. The teacher's lounge has such good cookies.

415. My wife feeds me well.

416. I bring home the money so I can eat what I want.

417. I don't want to share.

418. The food industry has made us addicts.

419. I am different.

420. I think about food constantly.

421. I am Presbyterian.

422. Baking makes a house so inviting.

423. I eat chips and dips when I watch television.

424. I am compulsive about everything I do.

425. I am an atheist.

426. I would have to go to a group and I don't like groups.

427. I wouldn't want everyone to know my business.

428. I am a Baptist.

429. I tried counseling and it didn't help.

430. God made me this way.

431. I have to study so I can't make healthy meals.

432. I only like meat and potatoes.

433. I don't like fruit.

434. I don't think like normal people.

435. Everybody eats like me.

436. I am Episcopalian.

437. I have potlucks with our friends too often.

438. I have the family over for homemade ice cream in the summer almost every week.

439. I have to have my coffee and doughnuts to get me started in the morning.

440. I love bagels and cream cheese.

441. Breakfast has to include bacon and eggs.

442. You can't drink on an empty stomach.

443. I have to have pancakes several times a week.

444. The extended family eats at Grandmother's every week.

445. My blood sugar gets too low.

446. Everybody goes to eat after church on Sunday.

447. My neighbor bakes and brings food over all the time.

448. I hate to throw away perfectly good food.

449. I eat ice cream by the half-gallons.

450. Well, I'm not an alcoholic like my father.

451. Hey, eating is a socially acceptable pastime.

452. My doctor is fat, too.

453. If I don't snack, I will get faint.

454. My grandmother was so fat and fluffy; I loved to be held by her.

455. I don't trust skinny women.

456. Men are too judgmental about fat women.

457. It has been in my family's genes, forever.

458. Sweets are my drug of choice.

459. You can't get arrested for being under the influence of sugar.

460. What else is always available and waiting, except my food?

461. My food doesn't judge me like people do.

462. My diet pills were taken off the market.

463. I have hypoglycemia.

464. Chocolate helps with my PMS symptoms.

465. My clothes shrink in the dryer.

466. Day-old bread is cheap and I can make cinnamon toast with it.

467. I am waiting until that new miracle drug comes out.

468. The gas station has all those goodies when I go in to pay.

469. The concession stands sell the best plastic-type cheese nachos.

470. I have to eat when I drink or I get too drunk.

471. The malls have all those food courts.

472. The company cafeteria makes the very best desserts.

473. Every day a different drug company brings food to the MD's office where I work.

474. What? Get together without eating? You crazy?

475. I ordered that stuff from the infomercial and it tasted awful.

476. I need a salt fix.

477. Pretzels aren't as bad as chips.

478. It is my mother's fault.

479. Amusement parks have such good hot dogs and cotton candy.

480. I ate fries and drank sodas for lunch everyday in the fourth grade at school.

481. The drink machines in my elementary school supported the free lunch program.

482. Sugar and caffeine give me a buzz.

483. I like food and the way it makes me feel.

484. I have to eat these foods to stay "regular".

485. I only ate a whole box of sugar-free cookies.

486. Sugar-free foods give me gas.

487. We are all going to die of something.

488. All of my associates are overweight.

489. America is a nation of fat people.

490. Sugar is a natural product.

491. If foods were really that bad, the government would do something.

492. Diet pills make me too irritable and nervous.

493. Low-carb or low-fat – even the "so-called" experts can't agree.

494. The magazines have all those tempting recipes and colored photos.

495. Even death-row inmates get to choose their last meal.

496. There are too many new restaurants in my town.

497. I can't hurt my grandmother's feelings by not eating.

498. Sugar is an energy food.

499. When I drive, I eat crunchy food to help me stay alert.

500. I went to one Overeaters Anonymous meeting and it didn't work.

Chapter Four

Your Excuses

1. _____
2. _____
3. _____
4. _____
5. _____
6. _____
7. _____
8. _____
9. _____
10. _____
11. _____
12. _____
13. _____
14. _____
15. _____
16. _____
17. _____

18. _____

19. _____

20. _____

21. _____

22. _____

23. _____

24. _____

25. _____

26. _____

27. _____

28. _____

29. _____

30. _____

31. _____

32. _____

33. _____

34. _____

35. _____

36. _____

37. _____

38. _____

39. _____

40. _____

41. _____

42. _____

43. _____

44. _____

45. _____

46. _____

47. _____

48. _____

49. _____

50. _____

51. _____

52. _____

53. _____

54. _____

55. _____

56. _____

57. _____

58. _____

59. _____

60. _____

61. _____

62. _____

63. _____

64. _____

65. _____

66. _____

67. _____

68. _____

69. _____

70. _____

71. _____

72. _____

73. _____

74. _____

75. _____

76. _____

77. _____

78. _____

79. _____

80. _____

81. _____

82. _____

83. _____

84. _____

85. _____

86. _____

87. _____

88. _____

89. _____

90. _____

91. _____

92. _____

93. _____

94. _____

95. _____

96. _____

97. _____

98. _____

99. _____

100. _____

101. _____

Okay, if you have more than this, you can use some different paper to keep writing them or use the margins. You can also add yours to the list of Excuses located at:

www.Overeating500Solutions.com

500 Solutions

Turn the book over to find the solutions. You have to do something to get something different.

The choice is yours.

Chapter Five

Your Journal

Your Journal

Your Journal

Your Journal

Your Journal

Your Journal

About the Author

Tonna Brock, M.Ed, MS, LPC is a graduate of Texas Woman's University. She has been a working in the eating disorder recovery field for 17 years. In private practice, she was the Owner and Director of Sherman and McKinney Family Counseling Centers for over 11 years. For three years, Tonna taught "The Survey of Eating Disorders" class at the Collin County Community College in their eating disorder counselor certification program.

For over 20 years, Tonna has been the main speaker at meetings, luncheons, workshops, retreats, treatment centers, seminars and conventions in the United States and Canada. She was the producer and co-host of a radio program, "Roads to Recovery" for several years.

Tonna is currently producing "KickStart Recovery Retreats", a weekend for overeaters to learn more about their disease and begin their lifelong recovery. She is also available for public speaking engagements on eating disorders and her "God as I understand Him" workshops.

Contact Information:

Tonna Brock, M.Ed, MS, LPC
P.O. Box 684
McKinney, Texas 75070

Tonna@Overeating500Solutions.com

Overeating?

500
Excuses

&

500 Solutions

Tonna Brock, M.Ed, MS, LPC

For information contact:

Skinned Knees Publishing
P.O. Box 684, McKinney, Texas 75070
Telephone 972 837-5102
SkinnedKnees.com

First Edition

Cover design by Lionel Vera. Layout by Pam Posey.
Printed by Hignell Book Printing, LTD.,
Winnipeg, Manitoba, Canada

Library of Congress Control Number:
LCCN 2005909373

ISBN: 978-0-9774420-0-3

This book is dedicated to the loving memory of
Joan Copeland Voss (1931-1976)
and
Roger L. Voss (1949-2002).

Acknowledgements

Everyone I have had contact with in my life has helped weave the tapestry of my life. My gratitude overflows when I think of my life today. I would write another entire book if I start listing individuals. I thank my wonderful children Myka, Mekala, and Luke, who have grown up to be people I love having as friends. (Now, that is another entire book by itself.) They have sacrificed much and loved so well. I thank Wayne, my husband and dance partner, for listening to my ideas and being my sounding board. To my father, Lee and my wonderful other mother, Doris, I give thanks for their prayers, encouragement and love.

My family of choice has been so instrumental to my growth and development. They believed in me until I could believe in myself. My "sisters", my Wednesday meeting, my women's spirituality group, my colleagues, and my friends have always been there for me in the good, bad, happy, and sad times. You know who you are and where we have been together. May we continue this journey for a long, long time together.

My teachers have been many. I am grateful for all of my clients and students who shared their lives, pain, joy, and struggles with me and I wish them well. Through the years, I have crossed paths with so many interesting, loving people at retreats across America. I think of you often with warm memories.

I love the saying, "If you had fun, you won." I did and I have!

Tonna

Table of Contents

Side A – 500 Excuses

Side B – 500 Solutions

Introduction

This is a book of 500 Excuses and 500 Solutions for overeating. Which side you choose to read is your choice to make. It is not your mother's, father's, brother's, sister's, spouse's, friend's, medical doctor's, therapist's, nor anyone else's choice. It is yours.

I have met many overweight people in my personal life and career. I have met very few who wanted to be overweight. Most folks would choose to be of a normal size. "Just push away from the table" we have been told. We think, "Who needs a table?" We eat in the car, the bedroom, the living room, inside, outside, anywhere, everywhere; the time or place makes no difference. We eat and we eat.

According to the World Health Organization in the 2003 Obesity and Overweight Report, there are one billion overweight and 300 million obese people in the world. Most of us may not know how many, but we know it is a major health issue. The Centers for Disease Control and Prevention states the known health risks: hypertension, Dyslipemia (a big, fancy word for high total cholesterol or high levels of triglycerides), Type 2 diabetes, coronary heart disease, stroke, gallbladder disease, osteoarthritis, sleep apnea and respiratory problems. But still, we eat and we eat..

There was a drug that hit the market several years ago. It was supposed to create a "feeling of being full". Therefore, overweight folks would simply quit eating. We laughed. Did the scientists really think we stopped eating when full? Did they ever listen to what a fat person really was saying? We eat when we are so full that we think we will explode. That drug was taken off the market because of side effects that resulted in many deaths and permanent heart damage.

I do believe there are some overweight people who do not understand the concept of calories and exercise. If a person

consumes more calories than she expends, she will gain weight. If he eats less than he burns, he will lose. Simple math. If someone eats or drinks 100 calories more than he needs every day for a year, he will gain over 10 pounds in a year. That is three-fourths of a can of soft drink, one tablespoon of regular salad dressing, or an extra teaspoon of margarine at each meal (100 X 365 =36,500 calories. There are 3500 calories in a pound.)

Then, the next year, it is ten more. After awhile, she decides to do something about it. Her medical doctor may hand her a "diet" or she goes to a dietician to learn how to eat healthy. She loses her excess weight and continues to closely monitor her weight. When she gains 3-5 pounds, she looks at where she is getting extra calories and reduces those or increases her exercise, thus losing the 3-5 pounds. This book may be helpful to those people.

However, I believe the majority of overweight people are compulsive overeaters. It is a disease. Food is a drug for them. Just as an alcoholic finds it nearly impossible to stop drinking, a compulsive overeater cannot stop eating. Oh, truthfully, we are great at stopping, especially on Monday and New Year's Day. We just cannot stay stopped.

Many of us have extensive knowledge about nutrition and exercise. Many of us have specialized in those areas, but to no avail. We are confused, frustrated, angry, sad, ashamed, embarrassed, humiliated, and frightened. We have tried countless ways and spent billions and billions of dollars, collectively, to lose weight and keep it off. There have been: bariatric physicians, diet clubs, herbal supplements, shots made from the urine of pregnant mares, speed, prescription and over the counter drugs, hypnosis, liquid protein, intestinal bypass, stomach stapling, stomach banding, liposuction, pre-packaged foods, jaws wired together, biofeedback, fasting, calorie counting, gyms, exercise equipment, low fat diets, low carb diets, clinic diets, high carb diets, diabetic diets, exchange diets, heart diets,

endless magazine articles and hundreds of infomercials. Most of them worked, for a while.

According to the American Cancer Society the survival rates of over five years for many cancers are currently greater than 90%. Of people who lose weight, 98% regain it within five years!

Once, I was at a public meeting where a woman spoke of once weighing nearly 400 pounds and her subsequent recovery. A medical doctor, who is personal friend, made an interesting comment after hearing her. He said, "With all the money that could be made by drug companies, there will be a drug developed that will allow people to eat but not gain weight." I stood there wondering, what about the obsession? What about all the hours spent thinking about food, eating food, preparing food, waiting in lines to buy food, cooking food, going out to get food?

The weight is a symptom of the disease – not the disease. Is it not like saying, "let's use an effective drug to reduce fever, but let's not worry about treating the infection that is causing the fever?" Guess what, the fever will spike up once the fever medication is discontinued because the infection is worse. Just like weight (plus interest) is regained by simply going on a diet, unless the addiction is treated.

This book is not about articles or research about nutrition, obesity, overweight, exercise, statistics, empirical data, or the latest facts. You can look up those on the Internet or in a library. You can educate and entertain yourself for hours. That could be a noble goal, to learn more and more. I am leaving that search for you, if you are interested. I have found "knowing" wasn't my problem, it was "doing."

What are the reasons or causes of overeating? There are many. Most experts believe the cause is bio/psycho/social (biological, psychological, and social. What is not covered under that broad area, except it being a disease carried by

UFO aliens?) We can all die of this while we try to figure out the cause. If we can stop, do we really care why we did it?

I promise you there is going to be nothing new or earth shattering in this book. Much of what you read here you may have already heard, read, or studied. I will try to give credit where credit is due. I've heard, but couldn't find the author of the quote, "All is wisdom plagiarized; only stupidity is original". There appears to be very few new ideas. Occasionally, I have come up with some brilliant, original concept. Then, I read it later in a book, written years before I came up with it. Drats, I hate that!

I admit I am prejudiced towards Twelve-Step programs. My personal recovery came as the result of working the steps. The steps originally come from Alcoholics Anonymous (AA). AA began when Bill W. met Dr. Bob in June 1935 in Akron, Ohio. According to a staff member at the General Services Office of Alcoholics Anonymous, as of December 2003, there have been 454 organizations that have been given permission to adapt the Twelve Steps[1] and Twelve Traditions[2] for their use. Obviously, I am not the only one who thinks they work!

Millions of people with all types of addictions, compulsions, diseases, issues, or problems have found recovery using the Steps and Traditions. We are all eternally grateful for the generous sharing of their program with other non-alcoholic organizations.

The purpose of this book is two-fold. It is to give you 500 Excuses and 500 Solutions for overeating. There are two lists, sometimes practical, sometimes ridiculous. It can be opened on any page and one or two ideas can be used. So, when you want to eat, there are 1000 things to read or do to not eat.

This is not a book written by someone who has just studied the subject, but by me, who has lived it, personally. I began my journey of discovery and recovery 26 years ago. I am

a Master's level licensed professional counselor so I have credentials and letters after my name. I started working in the eating disorder field over 17 years ago and have been in private practice for 13 years. However, most of my wisdom has come from skinned knees and elbows.

My intent is to write this book like I am talking to my reader. I have put inner-thoughts in parentheses because that is the way I talk. Sometimes, I take the scenic tour to tell a simple story. I will try to refrain from using multiple "!!!!!!!!" but that is how passionate I get about many things.

I watched my mother and brother die from overeating. I want to do whatever I can to prevent another compulsive overeater's death. My hopes are that this book will give you ideas to help you develop a lifestyle instead of continuing to live a "deathstyle".

As you will notice, there are actually two books you are holding. 500 Excuses and 500 Solutions. You decide which one you want to read. If you start in the 500 Excuses, you are the one who will have to turn it around to read the solutions. You can stay in the Excuses.

I had to *do* something different to *get* something different. I learned that, if everyday I went home and made my brownie recipe when I opened the oven door, there would be a pan of brownies. I could not make the recipe and expect there to be a pan of cornbread when I opened the door. If I wanted to make cornbread, I would use some of the same ingredients but have to change some of them. If I want things to be different in my life, I have to change some of the things I am doing. For me, not making my brownie *or* cornbread recipe was a start.

500 Excuses or 500 Solutions.

It is your choice.

[1]The Twelve Steps of Alcoholics Anonymous

1. We admitted we were powerless over alcohol- that our lives had become unmanageable.

2. Came to believe that a Power greater than ourselves could restore us to sanity.

3. Made a decision to turn our will and our lives over to the care of God as *we understood Him.*

4. Made a searching and fearless inventory of ourselves.

5. Admitted to God, to ourselves, and to another human being the exact nature of our wrongs.

6. Were entirely ready to have God remove all these defects of character.

7. Humbly asked Him to remove our shortcomings.

8. Made a list of all persons we had harmed, and became willing to make amends to them all.

9. Made direct amends to such people wherever possible, except when to do so would injure them or others.

10. Continued to take personal inventory and when we were wrong, promptly admitted it.

11. Sought through prayer and meditation to improve our conscious contact with God *as we understand Him,* praying only for knowledge of His will for us and the power to carry that out.

12. Having had a spiritual awakening as the result of these steps, we tried to carry this message to alcoholics, and practice these principles in all of our affairs.

[2] The Twelve Traditions of Alcoholics Anonymous

One – Our common welfare should come first: personal recovery depends upon A.A. Unity.

Two – For our group purpose there is but one ultimate authority – a loving God as He may express Himself in our group conscience. Our leaders are but trusted servants: they do not govern.

Three – The only requirement for A.A. membership is a desire to stop drinking.

Four – Each group should be autonomous except in matters affecting A.A. as a whole.

Five – Each group has but one primary purpose – to carry its message to the alcoholic who still suffers.

Six – An A.A. group ought never endorse, finance, or lend the A.A. name to any related facility or outside enterprise, lest problems of money, property and prestige divert us from our primary purpose.

Seven – Every A.A. group ought to be fully self-supporting, declining outside contributions.

Eight – Alcoholics Anonymous should remain forever nonprofessional, but our service centers may employ special workers.

Nine – A.A., as such, ought never be organized: but we may create service boards directly responsible to those they serve.

Ten – Alcoholics Anonymous has no opinions on outside issues; hence the A.A. name ought never be drawn into public controversy.

Eleven – Our public relations policy is based on attraction rather than promotion; we need to always maintain personal anonymity at the level of press, radio, and films.

Twelve – Anonymity is the spiritual foundation of all of our Traditions, ever reminding us to place principles before personalities.

My Story – The Recovery

This is the story of my recovery. The story of my disease is located on the other side of this book. I have heard many stories in my lifetime. Many I have long forgotten, but I know I learn from every story I hear. Some stories have changed my life forever and have altered my perception of the world. I am going to tell my story in chronological order and there may be random things thrown in occasionally. My life and my recovery happen that way.

I went three times in January 1979 to a Twelve-Step recovery meeting. (There are 454 different Twelve-Step Programs.) It was located in another town, seven miles from my home. I rushed back to my fourth meeting in October 1979. (In honoring the Eleventh Tradition, I will not mention which of those Twelve-Step organizations I have attended or been a member of.)

I was desperate. My high school reunion was coming up in June and I knew I couldn't lose all the weight in 2 months. I would have done nearly anything they told me in order to lose weight. If they had told me to stick my foot in the commode and flush it three times a day, I would have tried.

A woman from my town was at the meeting. She asked if I would help her start a meeting in our town. I said, "Yes". I knew this was a "rest of my life deal". I came home and told my husband. He said, "You don't have time to start a meeting. You have to take care of the girls." (Today, I get as much done in about an hour as I did in a week before the program.)

Literature

I read all the literature, which at that time wasn't much. I had my copy of the <u>Alcoholics Anonymous</u>[1] (the Big Book) and the <u>Twelve Steps and Twelve Traditions of Alcoholics Anonymous</u>[2] (the 12 &12). It said, "Half measures avail us nothing". Not 50%? No, nothing.

Step One

Step One talked about admitting being "powerless". (The Step and Traditions are located at the end of the Introduction of this book for your reference.) If you read My Story - the Disease, you can see that was a no-brainer. I had some problems admitting my life was unmanageable. I was good at managing my life and I could manage yours and everyone else's who would let me. I frequently even had a "Honey-Do" list for God, just in case He forgot who needed to be healed, needed a new job, needed to be protected, and on and on and on.

Sponsors

The group said, "Get a sponsor." What was that? I wondered. I was told it was to be someone who had what I wanted and ask her how she got it. I looked around and found no perfect people. I did find some people who had lost weight but I couldn't call them because I might bother them. A girl from another town called and said she was going to the original meeting I had attended. She heard about me and I was the only person who wasn't a long distance phone call away. We decided to sponsor each other through this. Talk about the blind leading the blind.

Food Plans

The group had a very low-carbohydrate food plan. Being the obsessive, compulsive dieter I was, I figured it out to have less than 60 grams of carbs and 700-2100 calories depending on your food choices. Of course, it was not necessary to figure this out, but I did. I was good at knowing about diets, going on diets, figuring the "hows and whys" of diets; just lousy at staying *on* diets.

I had to start eating three meals a day when most days I had only had a soft drink for breakfast. Now in the mornings, I ate 2 wieners with mustard and a half-cup of pineapple. I loved

barbequed chicken, so I would pre-cook several pieces on the grill and heat two for lunch and two for dinner. I stayed on it for 17 days and lost about 10 pounds.

Then, I went on a trip to visit Grannie. She was so very proud of me; she kept bragging on me. She had my very all-time favorite cake baked for me. The first day, I abstained. The second day, I had three pieces. The third morning, I started the day with a piece.

Grannie said, "I knew you weren't going to be able to stay on your diet." I considered pushing her wheelchair into the middle of the freeway. Then she said, "Please take the leftover cake home with you because I know how much you love it." "Not no, but Hell No", I said.

On Monday I started again. The goal was to abstain or be abstinent from compulsive overeating. My husband and I had birthdays to celebrate. I wanted to go to a steak house because I could get a small steak, salad, and a steamed vegetable; he wanted Mexican food. I thought about it and decided he should not have to sacrifice his wants and needs because I had a problem with eating.

I turned it over to my Higher Power and discussed it with my sponsor. I can still remember the amazement I felt at dinner. I found a dish that had meat cooked with tomatoes, peppers, onions, and yummy spices. The waiter didn't even flinch when I asked to substitute a salad for the beans and rice. The chips fell out of the basket onto my plate and I put them back in and not into my mouth. First obstacle overcome!

Since Thanksgiving was coming up, I kept asking other people what to do and planning my strategy. Some said to eat one serving of everything except bread, potatoes, and dessert. Okay, I could do that. As the day got closer, I spent much time worrying and re-planning the meal.

Finally, I decided to eat turkey, green beans, and a pickle. I felt satisfied afterwards but family members were rolling on the floor moaning about how over-full they were. As I walked home from my in-laws, I made a victory sign, "Da -da –da- du!"

Meetings

Our group held its first meeting on the first Wednesday night in November in a bank's Community Room. We had an article about our group printed in the newspaper and had 27 people that first meeting. Then, 27 different people the second Wednesday and 5 the third meeting! But, hey, it was the night before Thanksgiving.

The woman who asked me to help start the meeting only came three times. It didn't hit me until 12 years later that I could have quit, too. Luckily, several others helped to keep that meeting going in those early days. It is amazing that others have recovered, in spite of me, and our fumbling around, trying to learn how meetings should be conducted.

Someone asked, "How long do you have to go to meetings." Once, I heard, "I **have** to go to meetings until I **want** to go." (I keep going every week I am in town to that meeting. There are nights I think, 'I would rather go home and put on my pajamas and read a book.' But then, I remember the slogan, "If I keep doing what I am doing, I will keep getting what I am getting." I like what I'm getting. So, I go to the meeting and I have never regretted it after getting there. After 26 years of meetings, I am still teachable and I learn so much from everyone in the meetings, including the newest of newcomers. I also had to learn, early on, not to argue with myself. I always lose.)

Self-Discipline

I got a copy of "Just for Today"[10] and developed a program for myself. I did two things I didn't want to do and getting out of bed didn't count. I began cleaning out 2 drawers or cabinets. My house got clean. I discovered an interesting fact. If I did what I *wanted* to do (i.e. lie on the couch, eat, smoke, read, not get dressed, etc., I was miserable. If I did what I DID NOT *want* to do (i.e. eat right, exercise, clean the house, get dressed, pay my bills, write the thank-you notes, etc.), I felt wonderful at the end of the day. I started wanting to do the things that made me feel good about living.

Step Two

I saw the program had worked for others so I had no reason to believe it wouldn't work for me. (If I worked it.) I took Step Two and came to believe that a Power greater than me could restore me to sanity. There was no question I was insane, with the crazy things I did with food. I had always felt I was "different" from other people and I damn sure didn't want you to know I was different so I faked it. I wouldn't even allow myself to think about going to counseling because I didn't want anyone to know how "sick" I was.

Step Three

Step Three talked about turning our lives over to the care of God as I understood Him. I think I was afraid of God and didn't want to turn my life over to *the wrath and punishment* of God. I had to study the word "care" for a long time. A friend said she thought God must be schizophrenic because one Sunday the preacher said, "God is loving and forgiving" and the next, "God is jealous and angry and will send you to Hell". (A fear of Hell works real well in Texas because we don't want to end up anywhere, for all of eternity, that is hotter than it is here!)

I heard someone talk about "teabag" Christians who only prayed when they got in hot water. I think that was me. I realized, I knew only what others had told me about who God was. I hadn't tried to study and find out for myself. I began a quest to find out more about different religions and spirituality. I have an almost insatiable desire to learn. Someone once said, "Religious people believe in Hell and are afraid of going there; Spiritual people believe in Hell because they have already been there." I didn't like it there at all and I don't want to go back.

Step Four

Step Four was about writing a "searching and fearless" inventory of my life. I don't know how fearless it was, but I would write and write. I would hide it well. (Being a sneaky eater taught me lots of hiding places.) Later, I would start writing again. When I looked back, I would stop when I was reaching a really painful part of my life. I wasn't conscious of doing that, at the time.

Step Five

Step Five was "admitting it to God, to yourself, and another" those awful, deep, dark, nasty, horrible, terrible, bad things I had done and thought. I kept looking for the sponsor who had the aspects that I wanted: blind, deaf, and terminally ill. I decided to take it 100 miles away and give it to a priest because I'm not Catholic. I thought of calling a total random number and asking them if they had some time to listen. (This was before we had Caller ID.)

We were going on a business trip to Las Vegas. I'd give it to someone in a program there, so I'd never see her again. I had visions of the plane crashing and the only thing that survived was the black box and my inventory. I could imagine the newspapers being full of several pages of my story. My solutions are much more frightening than any of my problems.

One day, I thought about my best friend. She certainly hadn't been perfect. She was very open about her mental breakdown and her wild past. I realized I loved her and it didn't matter to me at all, what she had done at 15 or 18 or 27. I wished I had her courage to be herself without caring what people thought about her. (I probably would be real disappointed if I knew how little time those people did spend thinking about me.) Later, I learned that other people's opinions of me weren't my business anyway.

I decided to "give it away" to my co-sponsoring friend because she knew I had *some* redeeming qualities and wasn't totally horrible. I told her about celebrating my anniversary on the wrong date for eleven years to protect my reputation; that was a big skeleton in my closet that was going to the grave with me. (Today, there is no shame around that, obviously, or why would I write it in a book for anyone to read?) There wasn't a single thing in my inventory that there wasn't a word to describe, so I guess I wasn't original in any of it.

There was a sense of relief afterwards. No, the heavens didn't open and angels didn't sing. But, I didn't feel the need to move without leaving a forwarding address and changing my phone number. She hadn't run out of the room screaming. She accepted me as I was. I <u>began</u> to accept myself that day.

The next weekend, I went to a program workshop and the main speaker was so honest and told major things about her life from the podium. (I wished I had told <u>her</u> my inventory.) That day, another woman said that every time she wanted to binge, she calculated how much it would cost her and she would put that much away to spend going to workshops, conventions, and retreats. (I could have gone to South America, Europe, Asia and Africa on how much I have saved!)

More Weight Story

I had 28 days on my food plan and ate a piece of toast while on vacation, so I had to start again. Well, Christmas was coming pretty soon and everyone knows all those goodies. So...... I had to unzip my size 16 jeans on the way home from the Ranch Christmas morning. I was miserable.

New Year's Day was fast approaching! Of course, we had a family lunch on the first and I had to wait until the second of January to start because the leftovers had to be eaten. I planned what I was going to eat: a diet frozen fish dinner, veggies and salad. I called my friend and committed to eating that and only that. The fish was terrible so instead of that I ate fish-shaped crackers. No, I didn't count it as an abstinent day.

She started her food plan on a Thursday afternoon at 4 pm. That was amazing! It wasn't a Monday, it wasn't even a morning! (Look at your watch – you could start your recovery at this exact moment!)

One day, after I had lost about 10 pounds, I had stopped to get some cigarettes. This old man turned and watched as I walked by. This thing was working. I found the age of the men who looked fell about 10 years for every 10 pounds I lost.

I stayed on the diet perfectly for three months and lost all of my weight by March. I was wearing a size 8. Feeling great! People didn't recognize me when they saw me in public. One person, who had only seen me once before I had lost the weight, kept trying to figure out why I looked so different. "Didn't you have blonde hair before?" I never told him either.

I remember going to a party in an Oxford blouse and slacks, very conservatively dressed. I felt so uncomfortable and

vulnerable, I stuck as close to my husband as deodorant. I realized I knew how to act fat but not thin. (Of, course, my life was mainly an "act".)

Quit Smoking

I noticed that I was getting wrinkles at age 28. I knew smoking caused wrinkles and lots of other things. I realized that I was smoking as rebellion. Now, wait a minute. I was smoking because I was mad at others and I was killing myself. That didn't make sense. Besides, I had no desire to kill off my size 8 body. I decided to quit. I was ready.

I was trying to learn more about God so I was reading a bunch of spiritual literature so I would know how I understood Him/Her/It. Somehow, it didn't feel right to have a cigarette in one hand and a spiritual book in the other. Every time I wanted to smoke, I would read something. I read a lot in the next two months.

I didn't want anyone who had suggested I quit to know that I had. I didn't want them to think they had had any influence on my decision. The only time I really wanted a cigarette after that was when someone would give an anti-smoking lecture. "I can't see how anyone could smoke. It is the nastiest, dirtiest, blah, blah, blah."

Occasionally, I would smoke when I felt compulsive and that was the least dangerous addiction because I knew I would not be a permanent smoker again. One day, I bought a pack and planned my smoking all day long. I had to wait until my husband was gone and the kids were asleep. I only had a small window of opportunity. I smoked two and jumped in the shower to wash away the evidence. Since I had not had any nicotine in quite awhile, it hit me hard. I sat down in the shower and wondered if I should pray to live or pray to die. Any time I think about smoking, I remember that moment almost 19 years ago.

Fondling Thoughts of Food

In a story in the Big Book[3], the writer said he "couldn't fondle the thoughts of drinking". I realized I needed to not think about how wonderful food tasted, how creamy, how cool, how smooth. I needed to think about sitting in the closet floor, crying because none of my clothes fit. That one paragraph has saved my butt (actually, kept it off) many times!

Off/On, Again and Again

My husband and I went skiing and I got off my strict, controlled food plan. I had bought the kids "guilt" food, things I had quit having in the house because of my diet. I was leaving them with their grandparents and they bought them lots of "love" food. I came home off my diet with a pantry full of wonderful goodies.

Okay, since I was "off", I decided to eat 2 of everything. (This still sounds like the disease but I promise the recovery part is coming.) Nothing had that "ooh, laa, laa". The vanilla wafers weren't as crisp; the crackers were too salty. Something was terribly wrong! I decided to eat 2 more of everything. By six o'clock, I was lying on the couch with a cold rag on my head. I felt like dying. I asked my husband to go to the store for some Pepto-Bismol®. He wanted to know what was wrong. I told him I thought I had that virus our friend had on vacation.

The next morning, I got back on track, until we came home from church at noon. I opened the pantry and started with 2 of everything again. I might as well wait until the next day, which was a Magic Monday.

Thus began my next year of off/on the diet behavior. I would do well from Monday until Thursday night. Then I would have "controlled" binges. I would go to the grocery store trying to figure out what to buy. I would no longer be able to buy three different binge foods because I was dieting

again, starting tomorrow, of course. Cheese crackers or vanilla wafers were a better choice than chocolate sandwich cookies and chips. I only ate once on Wednesday since that was my meeting night. That time I didn't realize what day of the week it was until I had already overeaten.

I had a calendar and I would place a big letter "A" on the days I abstained from compulsively eating. Sometimes, I would have a string of two weeks before I would fall off the wagon or rape the refrigerator. Miracle of miracles, I was able to maintain my weight loss for the first time in my life. Sure, there were mornings when I had to lie on the bed to zip my jeans, but I had the weight off.

I remember going out to eat with friends. I was not going to eat any bread. I would sit watching it in the basket. "Well, I'll only have half a piece. No, I won't. I'll not put any butter on it. Oh, no, there is only one more slice in the basket. Now is my only chance because we are getting ready to leave." Sometimes, I would eat it and others I wouldn't. But, I could tell you who ate how many pieces and how they spread the butter on it, side to side or in a circle. I was so obsessed with the food, I was oblivious to my other surroundings. I learned if I have to talk myself into it, it usually isn't something I need to be doing. However, in the beginning, I usually lost the debate.

I learned there are five food substances that appear to be addictive: sugar, salt, white flour, caffeine and fat. I may have binged on a bag of oranges one day but I usually didn't six days in a row. Ice cream = fat and sugar. Cake with icing = flour, sugar, and fat. Pizza =flour and fat. Chips, fries, or nuts = fat and salt. Chocolate candy = caffeine, sugar and fat. Yep, that was my deal.

Goodbye Letter

Someone suggested writing a "Dear John" (breaking up) letter to food. I wrote,

Dear Food,

I loved it when we first started seeing each other. It was so much fun in the beginning, but lately, I feel so guilty afterwards. I am afraid people are going to see us together and so I have sneak around to be with you. I spend so much of my time obsessing about when and where we can meet next; I can't think about anyone or anything else. I know this relationship is going nowhere and I am only going to get hurt. I have to end this, even though I feel my heart is breaking because you are going to lead to my death. I want to love me more than I do you, dearest food. Goodbye, sweet, sweet, lover.

Love, Tonna

Clothes

I could wear fashionable clothes and not the old, fat lady styles. I felt wonderful - young and cute. I had on leotards and running shoes and was dancing to rock music when my husband came home for lunch. He said my attitude stunk. My five-year-old told me the microwave door wasn't a mirror. I was usually looking in the mirror to see if the weight had reappeared. Also, as I lost weight, I realized I was going to have the same body, only smaller. I wasn't going to be 5'7" and have long, lean legs, a concave stomach and a wonderful dark tan. Darn, I hated that discovery!

I needed new clothes. My mother had picked out or made most of my clothes when I living at home. Then, I had spent ten years wearing only things to cover me up. I didn't know how to make decisions. I took two friends shopping with me so they could tell me what made me look the thinnest. One outfit one friend liked the other didn't. The next one it was reversed. I looked over there at them. One was dressed in plaid and denim and the other looked like she could have been a hooker. Oh, my gosh! I learned other people's opinion and seventy-five cents would buy me a diet drink.

A friend had a group of women over and a fashion consultant talked to us. She said decide what style you wanted to wear, sporty, tailored, smart, and buy only clothes that fit that style. I wanted to be all of those. Also, to spend most of your clothing budget on the clothes where you spend the most time. I certainly didn't want to buy clothes for my kids to spill orange drink on.

I went and bought clothes I liked and I dressed like I wanted to look. I showed another friend my new clothes and she said, "Wow, those are sexy." No, I thought they were more glamorous. I thought about her statement. I realized I wasn't dressing for other women's or for men's approval. I was dressing for me.

Looking back, I had a period of wearing tight and youthful, the latest fashion, a glamorous stage, and a professional period. I think I had to go through all the developmental stages I had missed when I was fat.

After I had the weight off two years, I got the courage to give my fat clothes to someone in my group who was in the losing stage. My husband saw me carrying out all my sizes 16, 14, 12, and 10. He said, "Don't you think you will need them again?" I said, "No." (I haven't needed them for 25 years.)

One was a really nice, expensive pantsuit. It had been a Christmas present from three years before. It was the largest size in the junior department. It had been too small and I was too embarrassed to take it back to exchange it; that would have been admitting how fat I was. After going to the meetings for four months, I finally was able to wear it. Three weeks later, I tried it on and it nearly fell off. I am not one bit sorry I only wore it once.

Emotionally Grow-up

Some folks say we stop growing emotionally when we start using our drug of choice. I was only three. I have had to

grow up. I needed a group to help teach me and re-parent me. Someone once said group is a place to "gro-up."

I had always felt different than other people and I tried everything I could think of not to let others know I was. It was a "bad" different. As people started sharing their lives in meetings, I realized they were different, too. Sometimes, people want to see me as different "good". I just want to be equal to my fellow man/womankind, not one-up or one-down. Today, I know everyone on this planet is different and that is not a bad thing. I know I am not worth less than anyone nor am I worth more.

I heard a prayer once, "Dear God, Don't let me see me as others see me, I am not that good. Don't let me see me as I see me, I am not that bad. Let me see me as you see me, that's how I really am."

Wanted and Unwanted Attention

I began to get attention from the opposite sex and I started to freak out. My husband and I wanted another child. I was happy to get pregnant because I loved pregnancy, nursing and being a mother.

One added benefit was that I could be safe without gaining back the weight. I decided that pregnancy wasn't a permanent solution and this was my third baby! I did what the program suggested and wrote about it.

I did another inventory and Fifth Step about my weight and men's attention. I remembered two times when I was 12 years old and I looked about 16. I was not fat but so much taller than my peers, I felt like an Amazon. A soldier flirted with me at the Laundromat where I was by myself, doing my grandparent's clothes. I panicked, ignored him and got out of there as quickly as possible. An older man (he was at least 16 years old) kept looking at me in a restaurant. I liked and disliked it at the same time.

(I have heard, when people look at us with "sexualizing" thoughts, on one level, we know it. That statement resonated. There were men who came up and put their arm around my shoulder and said, "Hey, baby, you look good tonight" and I felt safe. Other men walked in the room, 200 feet away and I felt like I had been mentally undressed and I wanted to cover up. I need to honor such feelings. I am not crazy.)

I immediately gained weight. I would do the gain 10 pounds and lose down to 135 and gain 15 and lose down to 135, gain 20 and lose to 135. So, 135 was my barrier weight. I realized every time I lost weight, there was an incident where some man flirted, looked, or said something and I quickly started gaining it back. I think I unconsciously thought I was "invisible" or at least was wearing a wallpaper dress so I blended into the background when I was over 135. I grasped the thought of how scared I was of masculine attention. I wanted it and I was so terrified of it. Then, I figured out that I was afraid of my reactions to their attention. I didn't have good boundaries.

I, then, came up with the bright idea that if I didn't wear makeup no one would notice me. Once, I was in the hardware store and the clerks were flirting with me. When I got in the truck, (Yes, all good Texans have owned a truck at some time.) I looked in the rearview mirror and realized I didn't have any makeup on. It really hit me that I was noticed if I chose to be noticed, and not, if I didn't want to be. It had nothing to do with the weight or the mascara. When I went out with self-confidence and an attitude that I was worth knowing, I attracted people, not just men. Now, if people don't think I am wonderful, they have the right to be wrong.

Step Six

I became willing to have my defects of character removed. I know I have the disease of compulsive overeating, but I had to admit I also have the character defect of gluttony. I want what I want when I want it and you'd better get out of

my way or you may have tire tracks on your chest if you try to stop me.

I had so much "will" and I had some power over my decisions and actions, but not when it came to food. If it was in the house, I had to eat it and if it wasn't, I had to go get it. Once, on vacation as a teenager, my mother, three friends and I drove 70 miles - one way- to a truck stop to get some binge food after midnight because it was the closest place open that late.

I had to look at my dishonesty, selfishness, pride, shame, envy, gossip, manipulative behaviors, my procrastination, my people-pleasing, codependent actions, and my judgmental attitudes (Today, I still get very judgmental about judgmental people. Dang! I am still a work in progress.)

I had to look at fear. I was so fearful. In the 12 &12[4] of AA, there is a part about fear being the chief activator of all my character defects; the fear of losing what I have or not getting what I want. I have come to believe that any time I have a conflict with another human being, one or both of us, is afraid of losing or not getting. I react differently to angry people than I do scared people.

I looked at my list of resentments. What part did I have in them? On many, it wasn't pride, envy, greed, gluttony, lust, anger, or sloth. I saw that I had many items where I had simply, not spoken up. I had not said, "No, Stop, Don't". I had complied and I resented others for times I had not taken care of myself.

Step Seven

I asked God to remove those "defects of character that stand in the way of my usefulness to others."[5] One I have asked Him/Her/It to remove is my defect of talking too much. It hasn't happened. I would truly try to not say anything, but out something would come. Later, someone would say that

they really needed to hear what it was I said. Maybe that "defect" is just my personality and it doesn't stand in the way of my usefulness to others.

Step Eight

Step Eight was making a list of people I need to make amends to, for things I had done. I wanted to see an old boyfriend I had hurt very badly and tell him how sorry I was. Of course, I wanted to do it in person so he could see how good I looked. God had other plans and I did it on the phone. Dang!

Step Nine

Step Nine is making those amends. I apologized for gossiping about a woman and not being truthful about it when confronted. I called a regional manager of a tire company in Arizona and told him I was sorry that I had lost my temper and yelled at him. He was just doing his job, even if it wasn't what I wanted him to do.

In the Big Book, it talks about how the alcoholic is like an actor who wants to run the whole show, arranging the lights, the ballet.[7] Well, in Tonnaland, the birds would sing, flowers bloom, people would always be kind to one another, life would be fair. If people would do what I wanted, I know everything would be marvelous, simply marvelous. Sometimes, I write the script, but do not give the people in my play the queue cards. I get upset with them for not playing their parts, saying what I want and doing what I want. (WARNING: Do not share this part with family members. They will call you on it and say rude things like, "You didn't give me my lines you want me to say."I know from experience!) However, the Democrats, the Republicans and everyone in-between have their own ideas how this land "should" be.

I had to start learning not to "should" on myself. I was amazed how often I would hear myself saying that word.

A friend said she set standards. I asked myself, do I? Where in the Constitution, the Bill of Rights, or the Ten Commandants does it say other people shall fold towels or clean up like I want them to? When someone didn't do what I wanted, I began telling myself, "Tonna, you have choices. Say something, accept it, or do it your way." That certainly started changing my relationships.

Step Ten

Step Ten told me to continue taking inventory and when I was wrong, promptly admit it. When I catch myself giving false information or exaggerating, I say, "Oops, I just lied." Most people don't even seem to notice when I say it, but I do. Abraham Lincoln is quoted as saying, "When I do good, I feel good; when I do bad, I feel bad. That's my religion." I learned that is true in my life.

Step Eleven

Step Eleven is about prayer, meditation and improving our conscious contact with God as we understand Him. (Her, It) I started reading daily meditation books. (I got compulsive about those and there are so many on the market today, so I limit them to three-a-day.) I started writing a gratitude list for five to eight things each day. When I first started it was difficult to think of any. Now, I can think of thousands, I'm sure, i.e. showers, dental floss, toilet paper, my family, my friends. (Okay, okay, that would be another whole book!)

I have a little notebook where I write the following every morning.

> "I am enough (or whatever affirmation I decide on for the day). Please fill my heart with the desires of Your Heart. I truly want to do Your Will, today and always. I choose abstinence (from compulsive eating), health, healthy relationships, love, joy, peace, and serenity. I go forth in love, joy, energy, enthusiasm and abundance. I am loved and lovable, precious and adorable."

Finally, My Membership into Program

In November, after I had been in the program for over a year and at maintenance since March, I heard the Traditions read at a meeting for the umpteenth time. I finally got it. (See, what a fast learner I am?) Tradition Three was "the only requirement for membership was a desire to stop overeating". WHAT? I thought it said, "a desire to lose weight and keep it off". Stop eating what I wanted when I wanted? I was getting very tired of fighting the urge to eat. Most of the time, I wasn't happy even at a normal weight, which is what I always had thought was the key to happiness. I was getting ready to put the fork down. But,..... not yet.

I looked around at the meetings. I saw people, whose lives were so much better than when they first came to meetings, but they didn't have what I wanted. It hit me that there were two things I could get out of meetings. Relief or recovery. **Relief** came from going to meetings, getting out of myself, not isolating, reading beneficial literature instead of romance novels. The Big Book stated **recovery** came as a <u>result</u> of working the steps.

A man came to speak at our struggling Wednesday meeting. He said he had been abstinent for two years. Something way deep inside of me believed that if he could do it for that long, so could I. That could have been my first real Step Two.

My Hardest Step Nine

The biggest, most emotional amends - the one I had put off to last - was the one to my stepmother. My Dad had married her two years after my mother died. It is a long story and there is no purpose in telling it. I felt she had done some very mean things to me and my family. So, she owed <u>me</u> more of an amends than I did her. I felt she had done overt wrongs and mine were more covert, talking about her and thinking about, but not doing, evil things to her.

28

After I had lost my weight, she had her stomach surgically removed to lose weight. Her doctor had told her she wasn't 100% overweight so he wouldn't do it. She told him she would either gain the difference or she would find another doctor who would do it. He told her he would do it since she was so determined. I had called her in the hospital to see how she was doing. She was very rude to me. I thought about sending her a candy-gram but I didn't. I did call Grannie and I gossiped about her.

I told my Dad I needed to make my amends to her. He said she would hang up the phone on me. I said it didn't matter, I needed to do it for me, not for her reaction back to me. At Christmas, the guys went outside. We were alone. I told her I was sorry for all that I had done to hurt her and she actually said she was sorry for her part, too.

In March, I told Dad I was coming over. He seemed awkward about it. Then, he told me she had moved out. He thought she would be back. I went over and shared with him. I didn't feel like rejoicing that she was gone. I saw my father was hurting. I shared some program with him. I knew she was one of us, a compulsive person. The next thing, a new car, a new house, a new husband, a new job, a new piece of jewelry, losing weight, was always going to make her happy and it never did.

I no longer felt responsible for running my father's life. Most family members felt it was their responsibility to tell everyone else how to live their lives so it was usually my job, too. He was a grown man and he was hurting. I am not sure about the day before, but I know since March 29, 1981, I have not found it necessary to eat sugar desserts or to binge.

I figured it out later that the promises of the program come after Step Nine[4] which is where they are located in the Big Book, not after Step One. Interesting! I also believe if I can do it, so can you. If I can have over 24 years, so can you. There

is a woman I heard about in California who has over 40 years of abstinent recovery. If she can, so can I and so can you.(If we don't quit and we don't die, that is.) I believe, if I keep doing what I'm doing, I will keep getting what I am getting.

This is a "one day at a time" deal. However, I, personally, know I have to do this the rest of my life, one day at time. I needed to shut the door on sweets and binges. I don't need to make that decision every morning because, one day, I might be weak.

Today, I choose not to eat sugar desserts. I haven't had one in over 24 years. Some people judge that as being ridiculous. "One cookie or a piece of cake every once in a while will not hurt you." It might not hurt me but I can't think of a reason that it will help me. Some experts preach that depriving ourselves from a food will set up a craving and it is better to eat everything in moderation. I have been deprived from eating rat poison and I don't have a craving for it.

The secret is that I have no feeling of deprivation. I have a feeling of FREEDOM. I no longer **have** to eat it. I no longer have to go out at night in search of my binge foods. I don't have to fight it – should I, should I not? I am free. I believe if I keep doing what I am doing, I am going to get what I am getting – positively or negatively.

I have thought about this concept many times. If there was a pill I could take and be able to eat anything, any amount of food I wanted and not gain weight, if I was guaranteed I would have enough pills to last me until I was 210 years old, if the pills were in a place - secure from fire, wind, water, if I had complete access to them at all times.....would I take them? I believe the answer is "no." I know my compulsive, obsessive nature. I would be thinking when, where, what am I going to eat next? I would spend most of my time involved in some activity of eating, cooking, shopping, cleaning, or driving from restaurant to deli to bakery. I would not be free.

I have thought 'what if I knew I was dying'. No, I want to die abstinent. Excess food affects my thinking and feeling. I want to be fully present to life and to others. I don't want "dreams of sugarplums" dancing in my head all the time.

Today, I bake for friends and family. I can have sweets in the house. I don't need to avoid the sights and smells of food. I am free. (I didn't make my favorite desserts until I had about six months of freedom.) Miracles happened when I made chocolate chip cookies for the first time after I was abstaining. My recipe made about 3 times as many cookies. My kitchen was clean before the last pan came out of the oven. It didn't take all day to make them. I didn't need to go get on the couch, nauseated because I had eaten so much raw dough and freshly baked ones.

A friend was doing some construction work on our house. He said, "You have got to be on diet pills. You are constantly on the move." Interestingly, sugar is supposed to be an energy food. However, when I ate it, it was like unplugging from life. I was back on the couch - very lethargic. Today, I am commonly described as "perky and energetic."

I am not a sugar crusader. I am not judging if someone can or wants to eat desserts. I don't feel I am superior nor am I getting extra points in life. I only know, for me, I am free. There have been so many foods that have been invented since I quit eating desserts. I haven't tasted them and I hope I never do. I am free.

According to the Center for Science in the Public Interest's Nutrition Action Health Letter,[8] the pounds per person per year of sweeteners, i.e. table sugar, corn syrup, and dextrose (not artificial) was over 150 pounds in 1996. I figure I have already eaten my share. I might be caught up in 2051. I believe, although I haven't done a scientific study, that there are 2 in every 100,000 compulsive overeaters who can eat sugar with immunity. The problem is that the other 99,998 of us are trying very hard to prove, we are 1 of

the 2. Today, I believe I am allergic to sugar; when I eat it, I break out in cellulite and fat.

Gratitude for Timing of Amends

In the middle of May, I received a phone call from Dad. My stepmother had been in an automobile accident and was brain dead. She died thirteen days later. As I sat at her funeral, I was so grateful I had made my amends to her, just five months earlier. She had two brothers who weren't on speaking terms with her at the time of her death, one for four years and one for eight months. The reasons seemed so shallow that day.

I would have thought I had many, many years to make my amends to my stepmother. She was only three years older than me. She was dead at 32 years of age. Because of my amends, I could honestly be emotionally present for my father during his grief.

My Food Plan and Nutrition Ideas

Since I was pregnant, I knew my usual 500 or 5000 calorie diet was not going to work. I asked my OB/GYN what I needed to eat. He suggested I start with 1500 calories. If I did not gain enough weight, I would need to increase it.

What? I had never eaten what a normal person was supposed to eat. I was bingeing or starving. I decided I would eat 300 calories for breakfast and 500 for lunch and 500 for dinner and 100 for 4 PM snack and 100 for evening snack. I would eat balanced meals with no sugar desserts. (Three slices of pecan pie a day might equal 1500 calories, but it wasn't nutritious.)

After I weighed and measured my food and counted calories for several months, I learned what serving sizes were. A serving of meat is about the size of my palm. I knew the level my cereal needed to be to in my bowl for a serving. If

I ate a heaping full bowl of some cereals, it was equal to 4 servings. Remember, when airlines served meals on those tiny, little plates that looked like doll dishes? Well, those are the actual serving sizes of food..

The food labeling on processed foods is very helpful, but sometimes, terribly confusing. A 20-ounce bottle of soft drink has two and one-half servings; however, most folks think that it is only one. The calories are given as 100 in an 8 ounce serving, not per bottle, which is about 250 calories.. If I had 2 bottles, that would have been one-third of my total days caloric allowance. That, by the way, is over 15 teaspoons of sugar per bottle. I had to learn how to convert grams to teaspoons. One teaspoon of sugar has four grams.

A super-size order of fries has about 600 calories. I thought a fast-food taco salad would be a good choice until I learned it had over 1000 calories and more than 75 fat grams. (The FDA's maximum recommendation for a 2000 calorie per day diet is 65 fat grams per day, which would equal 48.75 grams for 1500 calories.) I looked up some nutritional information on the Internet to verify my facts. I saw one fast-food restaurant's salad listed for 340 calories which sounds like a good meal. However, lower on the list, it gives the calories for the croutons and the dressing, which raised the calories to 690 - if you eat it, as it is served. There are 415 calories of fat or over 46 grams. However, the big bacon hamburger had 580 calories and "only" 29 fat grams. Yikes, no wonder I was fat!

Many national chain restaurants have their nutritional guides, which include calories and fat available in the store (You may have to ask for one. Many times the managers report being out of them.) or online. It makes very interesting reading matter. I can also plan ahead, knowing what I will eat when I eat at each place. Ignorance may be bliss, but denial can cause my clothes to shrink!

A half-cup of pasta or rice is a serving, but some restaurants serve as much as four times that much. Of course, we don't

want to go to a restaurant and pay $7-12 for an airline size plate. Nowadays, a plate of food looks more like a platter enough for a family. The actual size of household dinner plates has also increased from 8 to 9 inches in recent years.

One good trick is to share a meal with a friend, but maybe order an extra salad. Another is to order a take-out box when my food <u>comes</u> to the table and divide it in half - before I start eating. I have another meal to enjoy later. (No, not as a snack, but another meal.) Whenever possible, I order low-fat salad dressing on the side. That way I control the amount I use. My taste has changed. I don't like lettuce swimming in a huge pool of dressing.

I find the more color in my food, the healthier it is. My lunch occasionally could be a cover-girl for a nutrition magazine. Baby spinach, red bell peppers, mandarin oranges with fat-free poppy seed dressing. Carrots and grape tomatoes. Sprouted grain bread (no added flour, sugar, or fat) with turkey breast, spinach, and fat-free mayo. What beauty! When I ate poorly, it was brown, tan and white. It is a no-brainer that the fresher foods are better for me than highly processed foods.

Sometimes in recovery, I have called in my food plan to my sponsor in the morning. I also have emailed a list of what I ate during the day to her in the evening. Sometimes, I have kept a small notebook and written down what I was going to eat after I had sat down with a meal. I may have ordered my meal, gone to the Ladies' room and written down 'I commit to eat only one-half of my potato and no rolls." No one ever noticed, except me and my HP. I am willing to try different things. If it works, great! If not, at least I am learning what does and doesn't work for me.

I had to learn to study food labels. The government requires companies to list the ingredients on food labels in descending order. I learned that to prevent listing the first ingredient as sugar, the manufacturer would use some of several sugars

in the product: dextrose, sucrose, fructose, corn syrup, and corn syrup solids to name a few. Tricky, eh?

My husband's company sent him to a well-known clinic to have a complete physical. The nutritionist gave him a meal plan and the MD's gave him a workout program to follow. He followed neither. Five years later when he returned for a follow-up visit, the doctors were impressed with the improvements in his cholesterol levels and his physical endurance tests. They questioned him about his lifestyle changes. He told them he had not done anything different. They said, "Something has to change to get this result." He thought a while and said, "Well, my wife went on a diet and lost weight."

He wasn't aware of the many changes I had made in our food preparation. I quit frying everything. I didn't put margarine in the vegetables. We had more low-fat ingredients. My changes made an big impact on my husband's health.

Luke's Birth

I began to have complications with my pregnancy and was hospitalized in Dallas. On the way to the hospital, I did my daily meditations. I realized I was powerless over when he would be born; I could only do what the doctors suggested. I felt so much peace being able to "turn it over to my HP."

Monday would be Myka's first day of kindergarten and I was in the hospital. My program friends came to my house Sunday night, washed her hair, cut her fingernails and got her ready to go. I didn't have to ask for help, they were there. The next morning, my son, Luke, was born two months prematurely. He was small, but in very good health. It was so difficult to drive away from the hospital without my baby. I told myself, "These are the most expensive babysitters he will ever have." He came home when he was 19 days old and had gained back up to 4 pounds 2 ounces. I had to feed him every three hours, around the clock, and it took an hour and a half to feed him. Mekala was almost three

and her nap time was when Myka came home from school so I could not nap. I look back on those days and I wonder how I managed to do it. I did it abstinent. Of course, there was always a load of clothes to fold and the dishwasher to unload. It all came to pass, not to stay.

Living Life without Excess Food

I knew how to live a life with thoughts and behaviors centered around food all day and night, month in and month out, year after year. I had to learn to live a life that did not revolve around food. It no longer took me 6 hours to go to the mall. Primarily, because I no longer stopped on the way to get donuts, eat Chinese food and a bean burrito, top it off with an ice cream cone at the food court and get two lemon fried-pies at the drive-thru on the way home, in addition to my three <u>diet</u> drinks. (Hey, that saved me about 1200 calories on three 32 ounce ones. That is 75 teaspoons of sugar or over one and a half-cup of sugar.) When I think about how much money I save by not practicing my addictions! I can go to an amusement park and not eat non-stop. I no longer run into the convenience store when buying gasoline and fill <u>me</u> up. (Some serve 44 and even 64 ounce drinks now.) I don't run through fast-food drive-ins for soft drinks and/or snacks. At restaurants, I don't purchase alcohol, tea, or dessert and often share a meal. I don't have to spend a fortune at coffee shops every morning.

Self-Care

I learned self-care. I got dental work done. I started having my teeth cleaned every six months. (Heck, I started brushing my teeth everyday, which I am not certain I did before program.) I go for yearly medical check-ups and mammograms. I very rarely have colds, flu, viruses which I had regularly when I was bingeing.

Being roommates with program women at retreats and workshops, I learned about make-up tricks, cosmetics,

electric toothbrushes, the best dental floss, nail polish, facials, and body massages. I have learned to respect my body and be a woman, not just an "it".

Diet Drinks

I drank a soft drink probably ever morning from the time I was 11 years old. Usually diet drinks because that counteracted the 6 donuts that went with them. Hey, look how many calories I was saving. I felt guilty because saccharine was reported to cause cancer. (My medical doctor told me I would have to drink 820 cans of them a day for an extended length of time to get the same dosage the rats consumed. I think 9840 ounces of liquid a day would kill me before the saccharine had a chance.) I drank at least 3 quarts a day. I loved them!

Over twenty years ago, the soft drink companies switched the formula to aspartame. The drinks were much sweeter and I wanted something salty to go with them. I knew it would take me at least two weeks to like them better than the saccharine. I decided to quit cold turkey. Of all of my addictions, I feel this one was the hardest for me to give up. Taking the returnable bottles back to the grocery the last time was like breaking up with a boyfriend. I would get up in the morning, put ice in my glass and open the empty cabinet before I would remember - I don't do that anymore.

Of course, I replaced them with a gallon of iced tea a day! I decided one day in 1989 as I was listening to a program audiotape while on a walk, I was ready to release caffeine. I believe that was also an act of self-care. Today, I occasionally drink herbal, decaf tea but primarily I drink water.

Once, my massage therapist remarked to my hairdresser that I had the healthiest hair she had ever seen. (Where I live was a small town.) They decided it was because I drink water and eat right. When a nurse gave me an IV, she said, "You have great veins, you must drink lots of water."

Alcohol

I continued to drink alcohol occasionally. One weekend, my husband and I went away for a little getaway. I had a bottle of wine and I liked how it made me feel. The next night, I decided to drive thirty miles to get another bottle. I didn't eat so I could feel the effect quicker. I knew this didn't sound healthy. I called a friend, who attended AA meetings, in the morning and told him that I wouldn't drink again until I called him. (Didn't want to shut the door totally.) Later, he moved and I didn't know how to reach him! I do not know, for certain, if I am an alcoholic but I do know I have a very addictive personality. If it feels good once, I want to do it ten, twenty times. I do know I can go anywhere and remember where I have been and what I did. I never have to worry about getting a DWI. I don't feel nauseated at night and yucky in the morning. Friends feel safe when we go out because they have a permanent designated driver. It has been almost 20 years since I have had a drink of alcohol. Hey, my friend has come back into my life so I could call him again. Nah, I don't think so. Today, I don't always know "what is God's Will for me, but I usually know, what isn't."

Since I don't eat sugar, drink soft drinks, alcohol or caffeine and don't smoke, what do I do? I just polish my "halo" and pat myself on the back!

Service

I guess I was doing service my first meeting because I asked another compulsive overeater to go to a meeting with me. Granted, it was for selfish reasons, I didn't have the courage to go alone. The Big Book states, in many places, that we cannot "keep it unless we give it away". Altruism is known to reduce depression.

I agreed to start a meeting in my town. I carried the key, the literature, I contacted the newspaper, sponsored many folks, disc jockeyed at the New Year's dance, made

buttons, created nametags, and taught line-dancing. I went to a Metroplex business meeting to help the groups in my area. Did I do it because I am such a nice person? No, I did it because I decided I wanted to live more than I wanted to die. If I have made a difference in one person's life, if I helped someone else get out of the Hell I was living, it has been worth every minute of my time.

I love to watch other people come into the program and begin their recovery. I get to watch first-hand miracles unfold. I feel like the stage mother who is bursting with happiness.

I think I served in nearly every capacity at the local and business meeting levels. I wasn't secretary because I still can't type. (This book was written by the hunt and peck method.) I learned Parliamentary procedure, how to conduct a business meeting, how to get things done by committees, (You take minutes and waste hours!) how to let go and how to teach others to do my "jobs". I learned that everything doesn't have to be "my way". I learned to love people who disagreed with me and my beliefs. I learned to look at all sides of an issue before making my decisions. I learned to listen.

I got over my fears of speaking in public as I read aloud the readings at the meetings. I was asked to tell my story at other groups, then retreats and conventions. Since I have lots of miles on my mouth, I am no longer afraid to get up in front of people. So, what if I am not perfect and make mistakes? I don't think I am going to die or have to move out of the country. I found out it was much more important to share from my heart than my head. I don't have to impress others. In fact, I remember making a deal with my Higher Power before I spoke the first time in front of a huge group of five people. If you want me to do well, I will. If I fall on my face, I guess there is something I am supposed to learn by falling on my face.

At one retreat in Colorado, I was given a button with "AFLE" on it. Miraculously, I have not made another mistake since that day. AFLE stands for <u>A</u>nother <u>F</u>-ing......(or fine)

Learning Experience. If something is a learning experience, is it really a "mistake"? A quote I really like that is attributed to Mark Twain is "Good decisions come from experience and experience comes from bad decisions."

I had never balanced my checkbook in ten years. I became the local treasurer and learned how to do it. I became the treasurer for the business meeting and then a seven state region. I learned how to get 501(C) 3 status for non-profit groups as I worked with the IRS for two of those groups. This was "big kid" stuff.

While giving service at the regional and international levels, I spent the night alone for the first time when I was 37 years old. (No, I wasn't scared but the opportunity had never previously arisen.) I learned to travel and manage airline reservations, frequent flyer miles, checking into hotels, renting cars and how to tip the bellhops.

I helped find an office for the business meeting. I was taught how to negotiate leases and contracts. I chaired a large, local convention and worked with hotel staff to arrange meeting schedules, banquets and breakouts. Later, I was co-chair for an international convention and spoke in front of 800 people.

I wrote articles for the newsletters, magazines and newspapers. Using a fictitious name, I did radio interviews. I was blacked-out like a mob informant on television to protect my anonymity. I worked with the media to get the program advertised.

I was the camp liaison at a retreat where the cooks didn't show up on Friday night, but the 57 compulsive overeaters did. The camp manager told us we could either cook the food ourselves or go home. We had a great dinner and lots of fun doing it. I learned that usually it is only the committee that knows what's going wrong and it is usually not going to be important in two years, anyhow. We had a banquet one year in a glassed-in atrium. It was twelve degrees in Dallas

that weekend. We had to eat our baked chicken breast while wearing our coats, hats, and gloves. We laughed about this being one banquet we would never forget and I haven't.

We had a Halloween party at a regional function. I made a program cheerleader costume - complete with sweater, a short skirt and pompoms. I realized I had never tried out for cheerleader in high school because I was afraid I would lose and I didn't think I could stand the rejection. (The next year, I was re-elected as cheerleader with twice as many votes, mine and a friend's. Of course, I had to vote for him, too.) We decided we were members of the 132 Club because on page 132 of the Big Book[9] it says, "We absolutely insist on enjoying life…..We are sure God wants us to be happy, joyous, and free."

Most of what I learned came with skinned knees and elbows. I heard on a tape once, "If I want to be criticized, do something or do nothing." I am not writing these things to brag on myself or pat myself on the back, but to tell you what a practical education I received by just being willing to give service and to learn. I learned much more in doing service in program than I did in getting a Bachelor's and two Master's Degrees. I didn't allow myself to say, "Oh, I could never do that." I couldn't until I did.

I went from being a very, frightened, little (big) girl who felt she had no talents or skills to being a very confident, successful human being. No better and no less than others. What I learned by giving has opened up so many doors for me professionally. I did it for free and fun, not expecting anything more than a stronger recovery. I came to program only wanting to lose weight and I have been given a life more abundant and fulfilling than I could have ever imagined.

I have friends from program from all over the United States, Canada, and many other foreign countries. I could call them any time I need help. I can talk to humans or answering machines or email them when I am happy, sad, mad, glad,

scared, frustrated, grateful or excited. I can share my victories and my losses. These are people who know about all of my warts and love me anyhow. I came and heard their stories and began to love them for being so honest and for trusting me. I told them about my most intimate feelings, and they loved and trusted me in return. I finally, slowly, began to love and trust myself. It feels very good.

Doing It Scared

One day a friend was sharing that she was going on an job interview and she was scared. Her sponsor told her, "Well, I guess you get to do it scared." Something inside of me clicked. It was a pivotal moment in my life. I had always "shamed" myself when I was scared. "You are a big girl (grown-woman) and you should not be afraid of_____ (fill in the blank)." I was so bossy and judgmental towards myself, no wonder I didn't want to be friends with me. I have probably never done anything in my life that I wasn't scared the first time I did it. Many of the things I even liked doing, after I got over being scared: roller skating, swimming, driving, dancing, parasailing, scuba diving, snorkeling, traveling in foreign countries, riding Ferris wheels. I found I need lots of courage to do things the first few times. Once I have experience, I don't need courage. So, today, I just give myself "permission" to do it scared or uncomfortable.

Shattered Angel

We had received a pair of glass angels that hugged a candle from my husband's grandmother's estate. One day, when she was about ten years old, Mekala wanted to have a candlelight dinner. I heard her open the hutch and I heard one of them shatter when she dropped one on the tile floor. As I came around the door, I saw a terrified look in her eye. I was able to go and hold her and tell her it was only an accident: she hadn't done it on purpose and I loved her.

I picked up the pieces and put them in the cabinet, not really knowing why, then I went back into the kitchen and continued cooking dinner. I was so grateful I didn't yell or lecture her on "being careful when carrying glass." The thought hit me, "Thank God for a shattered glass angel rather than a shattered real angel." I realized I felt horrible when I broke anything because I thought everything had more value than I did.

A few days or weeks later I read something about a woman who had a beautiful vase. She loved the texture, shape, color, but it was worthless because it had been broken and glued together again. I got out my glue and the shattered angel and glued her back together. There is a piece missing and her wing is chipped but she sits on my mantle. She represents a victory when I didn't shame my child. I don't know where the unbroken one is today.

I realized my life was shattered when I got to program. I believe the unconditional love of the people in Twelve-Step meetings and my Higher Power have put me back together again. I have stretch marks and parts that will never be perfect, but I have internal value. After sharing this story, friends started giving me angels. I have many of them. They represent solid love. People say they think of me when they see angels. I am glad I don't collect cows or pigs.

Stay Home Mom

We had decided that once we had children that I would be a 'stay home Mom'. If my kids ended up screwed up, I wanted to be the one who did it. I have heard "If it is not one thing, it's your mother". I think Moms get blamed for most of what wrong and Dads the rest. We all need someone to blame, unless we want to take responsibility, that is. Today, I believe most people are doing the best they can with the knowledge they have. Some of what they do is not good enough and some of it is. The problem is that we are usually just guessing at being a parent. We are

doing everything like our parents did or 180 degrees the opposite when the middle might be normal. (I have heard someplace, somewhere; The only "normal" is a cycle on the washing machine and the dishwasher.) I have never heard a parent say, "I wake up every day and try to think of ways to mess up my children's lives." I have heard there are four functional families in the United States. I have scouts trying to find them, but to no avail. They must be hiding somewhere.

Being a 'stay home Mom' is the hardest job I have ever done. I washed clothes and felt so good it was finally done. Thirty seconds later, there was another load of dirty ones. I felt like someone had nailed my foot to the floor and I had run around in circles all day long. Many in our culture do not value the job we do. We get no raises or performance reviews. The pay and 401(k) programs are non-existent.

However, I would do it again in a heartbeat. The rewards are invaluable. The joy and the fun of watching those little, annoying creatures grow into terrific humans are so wonderful. Those years go by so quickly.

If you read My Story – The Disease, you will have an example of the magnitude of how my overeating has affected my life. My children have not seen me overeat like that. Thank God they haven't had to experience me in my raging disease. They would probably tell you I can be controlling, but if they only knew what I used to be like. (I don't personally know anyone who isn't controlling, either passively or aggressively.) I don't think we have any followers in our family, just bosses.

My Purpose Here

Once, when I was reading a book, something was triggered. I occasionally get more from reading between the lines than I do the actual text. I had flash of insight. I had believed a high school diploma would make me a success. No. Well,

then a Bachelor's. No, didn't feel it. Teaching school? No. Master's Degree? Sorry, that didn't do it either. Success was a carrot I had spent over 35 years chasing. I couldn't seem to ever grab it.

I realized I was already a success and I didn't need to do another thing to be successful. I believe my purpose on earth is to develop a relationship with God, which I found through working the Twelve-Steps; done to the best of my ability today. To love others, which I do to the best of my ability today. And to change toilet paper rolls. I think I may be one of the very few living Americans who know this ancient secret. Whenever I see an empty roll, I take it as a sign that God has more work for me to do.

I don't think my address, my income, my career choices, my retirement fund, my education, or my degrees will matter in the end. I think the question on the final will be "How well did you love?"

My Philosophy

In case anyone wants to completely transform the world overnight, I believe the answer for everyone is to truly love themselves. Not the narcissistic, I am queen/king mentality, but a humble, self-knowing type of self-love. When we love ourselves, we don't want to be involved in behaviors that don't feel good. These include: anger, rudeness, selfishness, stinginess, rage and _____ (fill in the blank.)

Think about what Jesus said, "Love your neighbor as yourself". If we took that literally, most of us would never have a friend! We would walk up and tell her, "Gee, your hair is getting gray and you look fat in that outfit. You did such an idiotic thing this morning." All that within 15 seconds of greeting her! I read that as meaning Jesus assumes we love ourselves. It doesn't mean we should love others more than ourselves, just "as".

Working Again

When Luke, my youngest, went to kindergarten, I went to work part-time. I decided I had enough wiping noses and tying shoes so I didn't want to go back to teaching kindergarten. I went to a local community college to take aptitude tests. I learned being a truck driver, nun or potato farmer wasn't what I was interested in. I could have become a brain surgeon but I would be sixty-five before I finished medical school.

An eating disorder center opened up locally and I was contacted about working there. I was the community relations and marketing person. I said, "You could not run hard enough to make me be a counselor. I can't imagine listening to people piss and moan all day long." I've learned never to say "never."

One weekend, there was a retreat for the former patients of the treatment center. One of my responsibilities was to pick-up the speaker at the airport and take him to dinner. Since we were both in recovery, we shared battle stories and intimate stories of our lives. After delivering him to the retreat center, I drove home. I began critiquing my performance. Dang, why did I tell him XYZ? I could have talked all day and not said THAT! I wish I hadn't mentioned ABC. What he must think of me? Then, I thought he had told me some pretty goofy things he had done. I wasn't judging what he had said, only what I had. I liked him.

Sunday, I picked him up to take him back to the airport. I told him what I had thought on the way home. He asked me if I wanted to know what he thought about me. I said, "No, it is more important what I think about me." (I have not found it necessary to call him in 17 years to find what he really thought.)

The next week I went to a community college to speak on eating disorders. The Vice-President of Academic Affairs

took me to dinner afterwards. We were the same age and we shared our life experiences with each other. On the way home, I thought, "He liked me."

I couldn't wait to tell my friend the next morning. My friend said, "It sure seems like you need people to like you." Well, that let the air out of my balloon! As I thought about that remark, I realized that was the first time I had ever gone somewhere and felt the other person liked me. I felt I always liked the other people more and they were only "putting up" with me. I can't remember ever feeling that way again. (Today, I am fun to be with, even if I am the only one that feels that way.)

I went to work for another treatment center and started helping with some groups and found I enjoyed it very much. I discovered many professionals did not know or understand the Twelve-Step programs and recovery programs that were available. I thought, "If the professionals don't know, then the layperson probably doesn't either." I wrote a letter to several radio stations and told them I had a good idea for a "Roads to Recovery" talk show. I was co-host and producer for three years. I met so many fascinating people and, again, learned so much.

Graduate School Revisited

Going back to school was an interesting experience. I found that I wanted to learn. When I went to college when I was eighteen, I only wanted to get a "piece of paper", not necessarily, to learn. I was dealing with my perfectionism. I decided I didn't have to make all A's. B's were good enough. The problem was I knew how to try to make A's or how to do nothing and make F's, but how much did I need to do to make a B. C's in graduate school didn't count.

In my first class, I had three research papers due. I wrote one. I looked at it. "Could it be improved, could I do more research? Yes. What was the purpose of doing the paper?

To learn about the subject, not to impress the teacher with my skills as a researcher and writer. Did I learn about the subject? Okay, turn it in!" The papers were worth 50 points each. I made a 50, 49, and 48 on mine. Golly bum, I would have spent so much more time obsessing on them.

I did not drive myself insane seeking perfection. I made all A's except in 2 classes. This disappointed me. The teachers didn't give A's in those courses and the semester after I took them, they went to a pass/fail grading system for those. Dang, I learned I am still not over my perfectionism.

I have never had a client come into my office and ask to see my transcript to check my grades. No insurance company requested my grades either. No one even knows or cares what I made in college. Why did I spend so much energy worrying about them in the past? (My Dad always reminds me worrying doesn't help anything. "Show me one thing it has changed and I'll tell you to worry." I know 99% of everything I have ever worried about hasn't happened, so I think it has to be highly effective.)

In one class, we had to do a poster. On the front of it, we were to cut out words, phrases and pictures to describe our 'self' we presented to the world and on the back, the same for our inner 'self'. I was very proud of mine, until I got to class. On the outside, I was happy, capable, dependable, responsible, hip, slick, cool, and able to do it all. Inside, I was terrified, anxious, knowing everything was going to fall apart any moment and people would know I didn't have a clue what I was doing. I was so good at faking. I wanted to go sit in the corner and suck my thumb.

The professor told us after we presented our posters to the group, "The goal in life is to be congruent; your insides match your outsides." Great, mine were totally opposite. But, wait a minute; I did pay my bills on time. I got my kids to school everyday with clean clothes, teeth brushed, and lunch money. I was responsible. I did follow through on

commitments. Maybe, the inside was the one that wasn't the real me. Today, I believe I have one of every age I have ever been inside of me. I think my five-year-old little girl has had control of my feeling states. It wasn't my adult who was scared to do grown-up activities. It was my little girl.

I didn't need to shame her. "You shouldn't be afraid to call the operator to ask how to do a conference call. You are a grown woman." I need to acknowledge her feelings and parent her as I would my children. "Okay, Tonna, I know you are scared and feeling shame for not knowing how to do this. I will go with you and we will make the call together. It is okay to not know, people will help you learn."

There is an old Alanon[10] saying – "I can do anything for the next 12 hours…" I have adapted that many times in my life. "I can take statistics for the next 4 months even if I would kill me if I had to do it for the rest of my life." (I ended up liking my statistics class.) I've thought about that many times. I could probably go out and stand in dog poop for 2 weeks, if I had to. Do I want to? No. I don't need to want to do things. I don't have to like it. Sometimes, I just have to do it anyway. I may have to do it scared, uncomfortable, or nervous. I just have to do it. Where did I come up with the idea I have to be comfortable 24/7?

In one course, we were to write six to nine page process papers on different subjects. Not research, but real life experiences. One I wrote about was "My Body – My Body Image." I realized that 99% of everything I disliked about myself had something to do with my body. It was my weight, the stretch marks on my breasts and hips I got in fourth grade when I developed too quickly, my breasts - either too soon, too big, too saggy. It was guilt about my sexual behavior, which was connected to my body. I am basically an honest person. Most of my lying had been related to sex or eating, which was related to my body. I have been struggling to accept my body "as is" since I was 6 years old. I look in the mirror and tell myself that this is what 54 looks like. I

don't want a face-lift. (Today, that is.) I don't want to look like someone else. I want to love and accept me as I am. My face maps my life. WARNING: If every man, woman, and child accepted themselves today, the economy would collapse. Think about how much we spend trying not to look, smell, taste, be who we are. Of course, the companies, who do not want us to be satisfied with ourselves, finance the media.

What Teaching Taught Me

I was asked to teach a college course, "The Survey of Eating Disorders" at a local community college. It was a required class for the certification program for eating disorder specialists. I went from teaching kindergarten to teaching college. Many of my students were licensed counselors getting certified, many were "returning" students in their thirties, some were fresh out of high school, some were interested in the subject and many were taking the course looking for help with their own eating disorder.

My students had an assignment to read and write a review on two books and then write a paper comparing them. One suggests becoming friends with all foods and never depriving yourself. The other takes an addiction approach and recommends omitting all sugar and white flour. It was interesting because the students who didn't have an eating disorder favored the "eat what you want" book and those with eating disorders felt the abstinence book was the better solution.

I would have my students write reaction papers on the speakers and activities we did in class. I couldn't wait to get home after class to read them. A speaker came to talk and the reactions were, "If I ever needed to go to treatment, I would want to go to that man. Another, "I wouldn't trust that man. He seemed like a snake-oil salesman." Another, "I learned more from him than anyone so far." Another, "He didn't have a clue what he was talking about." Those were about the same speaker. I found by the end of the semester,

I could predict who was going to like the speaker and who wasn't. I based my predictions on their previous reactions and from their individual belief systems.

Why didn't everyone agree? I really thought about that one! I decided I could give a person a list of 30 people to interview and ask their description of me. This is what you are likely to hear:

- One of the most spiritual and loving people in the whole world
- A Bitch
- A real "Can Do" person – if you want it done, call Tonna
- Quite and shy
- Has to be center stage all the time
- Lazy
- A workaholic
- A brilliant, intelligent person
- I don't know how she manages to get to work. She's dingy.
- Perky and energetic
- Too religious
- A real wild heathen

Which of those am I? I am the loving and spiritual one, of course. (I like that one best). Actually, I probably have all those facets. I can also tell you who would say which of those. Who is speaking determines what is said. The smart one thinks 'I'm dingy'. The dingy one would say 'I'm smart'. The wild ones would say 'too religious' and the religious person would say 'I was wild'.

I could ask you to describe former President Bill Clinton. When you finished, I might not know about him, but I would know about you. I would know if you were Democrat or Republican, big or small government, what you believe and value. So. I know I had better be careful when talking about others because I am defining myself.

God As I Understand Him Workshops

I started doing "God As I Understand Him" workshops. The ideas and parts came to me from various things I had done and participated in throughout the years. It is a synthesis and has evolved. I have been privileged to be able to facilitate many of them throughout the United States. I loved doing them so much I went back to college to get a Master's degree in Counseling and Development so I would have the correct letters after my name to open doors.

I have done the workshops with groups that were mostly Baptist, Methodist, Catholic, Mormon, Jewish, New Age, Episcopal, non-denominational, and have had Hindus and atheists in attendance. It has been amazing to me how similar the results have been in each group.

The purpose of the workshop is to explore our relationship with God as a child, as an adolescent and young adult, and to decide what we want it to look like today.

Most people see God in the same image of their earthly father. If their Dad was available, distant, punishing, absent, abandoning, loving - this is how they see God. Some literature discusses a person's concept of God as self-referencing. They create God in their own image. I see both ideas in people's discussion. Some folks say God is very punishing and is going to send you straight to Hell. They would be glad to personally buy you a one-way ticket because they are so judgmental. (I still get real judgmental about judgmental people! Dang, I don't like that defect of mine.) Some don't ever see God forgiving them and they never forgive themselves. Those who feel God is "there" for everyone else, but not them – they are never "there" for themselves.

I decided the topic of my professional paper would be "God as I understand God: A Handbook for Counselors" and I told the Chair of my committee that I wanted to graduate that May.

She said that it takes more than one semester to get it written, corrected, typed in the proper format and bound. I said I would get it done. I had all those memories of procrastinating for 5 years on the first Master's. I did it in time.

Licensed Professional Counselor

When I completed my course work, I had to have 2000 hours of supervised training before taking the exam to get my License as a Professional Counselor. Most of the hours are done on a volunteer basis. It is real luck to find somewhere that actually pays interns. I sat down and wrote exactly what position I wanted to have. I immediately ran out applying for jobs people recommended to me, none that I wanted.

I remember being so disappointed I wasn't offered a job I absolutely knew I didn't want. Of course, I would have probably taken it. Three months later, I looked around my office and I was doing exactly what I wanted to be doing.

My supervisor was in private practice and I was doing contract work. She decided to do an internship in Canada and asked if I wanted to purchase her business. I was terrified of getting a loan and doing "real big kid" stuff. Someone asked me, "How scared are you going to be if you don't buy it?" Well, I wouldn't have a job.

I did it scared. I had two offices and contracts with many insurance companies. All the skills I had learned though service in my recovery program were really training for my paying job! I could negotiate office space, do marketing, understand financial statements, and much more.

I have learned so much from my many clients who have opened their lives and allowed me the sacred honor of being present as they heal. There is so much pain and hurt. I feel that what got most people to my office (besides their vehicles) was having two conflicting feelings at the same

time. She loved and hated him at the same time. He wants to leave and to stay at the same time. I have never had any client who could honestly say he/she loved him/herself.

After eleven years of being a business owner, I recently sold my two offices. I plan on continuing to see current and former clients. One couple recently remarked, "We like to come in for our 10,000 mile check-up every couple of years."

People often ask me "How can you stand listening to people's problems all day long, day after day." I found I love it and I love my clients. I can do it because I have hope for each one's healing –sometimes they heal quickly and sometimes slowly. As long as there is breath in their body, I will have hope. I have been privileged to watch as people experience change in their lives.

Woman's Spirituality Group

A friend of mine and I experienced some major spiritual abuse in organized religions. We felt we needed a sacred space to explore our spirituality. A woman's group was started twelve years ago. Most have been in various Twelve-Step programs. We have laughed, cried, disagreed, rejoiced, supported and loved each other.

Our group has been fluid with women moving in and out of the group. It has been a wonderful experience for me to learn to trust women. We don't have much contact with each other during the week, but we know we are there anytime for each other. We have met in homes. There is no money collected. We are not "guilted" for lack of attendance or service. We show up and we are always welcomed. We are honored and not judged. There isn't competition among members. There are no power struggles. We believe in each other and we experience the joys and miracles in each other's lives.

We have started many books and have finished a couple. We each have a freedom to explore different ideas and

share them with the group. We have tried many different ways of expressing our spirituality.

We sit in our sacred circle and hold hands as we close. We ask each other to believe for us what we have difficulty believing for ourselves. It is a known fact that every week I am going to ask God for healthy relationships. (I have them today. I am eternally grateful and I certainly enjoy them!)

Divorce

I had known for a long time I wasn't happy in my marriage. I would pray for God's Will and for God to change my heart about wanting a divorce, for many years. It was never in my script for me to be divorced. Cinderella had "lived happily ever after". Life would be so much simpler without dividing the Christmas decorations and family photos. I tried to figure out how it could be done without hurting anyone, without costing money or financially burdening us and our children, without me wearing the black hat, and I couldn't do it. I didn't want to be a bad example for my children and others.

I am not going to write my reasons for wanting the divorce. My ex-husband is the father of my three beautiful children and a very decent human being. Suffice it to say, I was 17 years old when I got married and I had no idea what marriage really was. I went from my mother and father making my decisions to my husband making them. We each came into the marriage with baggage and we each were just guessing at how to have a relationship.

I told my husband over six years before I left that we had to do something different or I was leaving. We didn't make any changes. We didn't go to counseling. I came to believe my husband didn't need to change because he wasn't what I needed. He seemed happy with who he was. We both grew up and grew in different directions. Today, I believe I slept in the same bed for twenty-six years with a man who didn't ever really know me nor did I know him.

My mother was told at 43 years of age that she had 6-12 months to live. I hit 43 and I asked myself, "You could only have 6 months to live, is this how you want to live it?" My answer was. "NO".

I had visions of my husband, my children, my family, our friends, the community, and God being on one side of the line and me, all alone on the other. I had to face the horror of telling and hurting my children. I grieved what "shoulda, coulda, oughta" been. I had to go to the edge and jump, not knowing if anything was there to catch me. I had never lived alone or been totally responsible for myself financially.

I jumped. I filed the papers and went before the judge without an attorney. The clerk was stamping the final papers and she said, "Congratulations". That felt wrong. I knew it was something I needed to do for myself to survive emotionally, but it wasn't a happy day. We didn't argue about the settlement. The divorce cost $167.

Myka was in college. Mekala and Luke lived with their Dad Monday through Thursday and with me on the weekends. My ex-husband and I have been able to cooperate and work well with each other for our children's sake. We have been through two weddings very graciously and I am extremely grateful.

Once, a person said, "Don't you feel you wasted those 26 years of your life?" No, I don't. It took every minute of my life to create who I am today. Had I made one different decision, I would have had a different result.

I can remember a period of my life when I ran around saying, "Who am I?" I am a mother, daughter, wife, but "who am I"? One day, it hit me. I knew who I was. I was sum total of all the decisions I had made up to that point in my life. The real question is, "Who do I choose to become?"

Dating

For two years after my divorce, I dated and developed a relationship with myself. I had known all of my ex-husband's favorites: movie, restaurant, food, style, color, singer, song, etc. Did he know mine? Heck, I didn't know mine. Today I know. (And, so do most of the people in my life because I tell them.)

My ex-husband got re-married. Mekala graduated and Luke had his own friends and life. I decided I was open to having a relationship. I did not have anyone ask me out until I made that decision and almost immediately afterwards, I did. Funny, how that worked. I wonder if I was wearing a sign "Closed" and I changed it to "Open". I figured I wasn't going to go into my living room and find a man sitting on my couch. If I wanted to meet men, I had to go out into the world to meet them. I did it scared.

I believe when we start dating again, we are the age we were emotionally when we stopped. I was 17. I would stand there, blushing, not believing what had just come out of my mouth. I was "gunky." I felt like a silly high-school girl.

I wanted to take dance classes. I had three friends go with me one night and I loved it. They weren't interested in continuing. I called everyone I could think of to go with me. No luck. I decided it was something I really wanted to do. The classes were in a nightclub. I was scared to go alone. I decided to take a sweater and I put it on the back of a chair. I ordered two waters and put one in front of the chair with the sweater. I thought men would think my "friend" was either dancing or in the ladies' room.

I discovered I could learn so much by just dancing with a man once. I could tell if he was respectful, a show off, controlling, sexually inappropriate, timid, or had any rhythm. I joined a dance club. I went to single dances.

I feel I learned as much in relationship with each one I seriously dated, as I would have in five years of therapy. All of my issues surfaced and had to be dealt with.

I had my heart broken by the first man I dated. We had been together for six months. We had so much fun together. His kids loved me and mine loved him, too. He sent an email saying he was going to try one more time to get back with his ex-wife. I had never had my heart broken. I didn't know a person's heart physically hurt. I hoped that one repaid some negative karma. I realized I had a choice. I could protect my heart and never be hurt again or I could give 100% and risk heartbreak again. I chose the later.

I learned that it is my love that hurts me the most. If I don't care, when someone dies or leaves, I am not going to hurt. The more I love the more I am going to hurt. I decided the joy is well worth the pain.

I learned all of my emotional pain is caused by me not wanting things to be the way they are at that moment. (It doesn't mean I can't do something about it in the next moment.) If someone dies, the more attached I am to the idea of them not being dead, the more I grieve. Huh, wasn't that what the passage about acceptance in the Big Book[11] was saying? (That I had been reading for nearly 20 years and had memorized) I had the information that was in my head, finally reach my heart. I *experienced* it.

One day, I realized a man I was dating had no living people who loved him. He didn't seem to care. I had always felt unloved but I knew so many people *really* loved me. I could make a long list of people who would do anything for me. I haven't felt unloved since that moment of enlightenment.

I had been dating one man for about a month. He told me he was afraid I was falling in love with him and he wanted to let me know he didn't have time to fall in love because he had a new job and his son's were a priority in his life. (When

I am in love, I still go to work and take care of my children and myself.) I was so happy! This man told me he was emotionally unavailable and I wasn't devastated. I wasn't unlovable and I did not have to "make" him love me. I felt like the wicked spell had been broken. I was free at last!

I thanked him for the information because I could make an informed decision. I had choices. I could continue to date him because I enjoyed his company or I could stop dating him altogether or I could date him but be open to meeting someone else. I continued dating him.

My Hardest Year

In 2002, I had the hardest year of my life. My only sibling died. I lost a huge contract that was the bulk of my business. I had neck problems and spent $6000 out-of-pocket on treatments that didn't fix the constant pain. I ended a three-year committed relationship. So, I guess I could say I had losses in my health, wealth, family and love. All the things I value the most in life.

The relationship breakup was in October. I was really sad the night we made the decision. The next night I came home very excited and happy. What I had realized was that I was going to be happy. I got it all the way down to my toes. I would be happy with him, without him, with someone else, or all by myself, because who I was in my insides was happy. The external events and challenges are not going to determine my happiness, it is internal.

Commitment

When Wayne and I started our relationship, we wrote a Mission Statement for our relationship. (Okay, We discussed it, I wrote it and he edited it.)

What was the purpose of our being together?

To treat each other with dignity, honor, and

respect. To encourage each other's personal growth. To practice the relationship skills we have learned, and to model to our children what a healthy relationship can be.

I am a giver and I want to give to the people I love what they need and want. I had always been able to read their minds about what they wanted. The problem is, that I expected them to read my mind and give me what I wanted and needed. It didn't count if I had to ask. Well, I learned I am not such a good mind reader as I thought and most folks I know aren't any better. I made a commitment to Wayne that I would ask in a clear and direct manner for what I wanted and needed. He's not required to figure it out on his own.

I have had such a hard time asking for help that a "no" was devastating. I would watch the person's body language and immediately say, "Oh, never mind, I'll do it myself" if I detected a millisecond of hesitation. I made a commitment to accept "Yes" and "No". If he doesn't have the freedom to say "no", he will never be able to say an honest "yes". If I were to get no's all the time I would need to re-evaluate our relationship. If he's in the middle of watching a television program and I want to talk, he can say, "Honey, not right this minute." I can call a friend or check my email or read. I don't have to have instant gratification. Interestingly enough, I don't get many "no's".

I made a commitment to be honest. This continues to build our trust account. I am honest more for my sake than for his. I don't like who I am when I am being dishonest. I trust him to tell me the truth. The mutual honesty feels so good. We don't have to remember what we story we told when we tell the truth.

Wedding

My partner and I decided to get married. We were going to go to the justice of the peace. On Wednesday night, I decided I

wanted a wedding because I hadn't had one the first time. (I hoped this was my last chance for one!) I had the woman's spirituality group coming to my house on Sunday afternoon so we decided to get married after it was over, when many of my closest friends would already be here. I called many others and our family.

I looked around in my closet wondering what I would wear. Wayne hates suits. We both had new warm-ups. I told everyone to wear warm-ups or jeans. Mekala asked me why. I told her we would have on running shoes and could get away in a hurry, if we changed our minds. She told me I was a freak. I love being weird because I can get by with such a wide range of behavior.

Luke and his future wife, Kerri, sang a duet. We had candles and roses. Here are our vows we made to each other.

Our Wedding Vows

This family, either by birth or choice is joined together this evening to be a part of the marriage of Tonna and Wayne. They choose to continue their life together as husband and wife.

Wayne, Tonna, please take your individual candle and light one of the wicks in the large candle to represent yourself in this marriage and then light the third wick together to represent the part of your life you will share. As you light this candle tonight, may the brightness of the flame shine throughout your lives. May it give you courage and reassurance in darkness. Warmth and safety in the cold. Strength and joy in your bodies, minds, and spirits. May your union be blessed forever.

Wayne, do you commit to continuing to treat Tonna with love, honor, dignity and respect? To be her playmate, companion, dance partner, snuggle buddy, lover, and friend, in the good times and

during life's trials? To accept her children, Myka, Mekala, and Luke, and her family as yours?

Tonna, do you commit to continuing to treat Wayne with love, honor, dignity and respect? To be his playmate, companion, dance partner, snuggle buddy, lover, and friend, in the good times and during life's trials? To accept his children, Marcus and JC, and his family as yours?

May I have the rings? Wayne, will you place the ring on Tonna's finger and repeat after me? With this ring, I, thee wed.

Tonna, will you place the ring on Wayne's finger and repeat after me? With this ring, I thee wed.

I now pronounce you husband and wife. You may kiss each other.

May your marriage bring you all the blessings a marriage should bring, and may life grant you patience, tolerance and understanding. May you need one another, but not out of weakness. May you want one another, but not out of lack. May you embrace one another, and let there be spaces in your togetherness. May you succeed in all-important ways with one another. May you look for things to praise and take no notice of small faults, remembering to say I love you. If you have quarrels that push you apart, may you both have the good sense to take the first step back. May you have happiness and may you find it making one another happy. May you have love and find it loving one another. May you be well, peaceful, and at ease. Thank You God for Your Presence here with us, and Your blessings on this marriage. Amen.

After the ceremony, I fed him wedding cake and he fed me a carrot. It was a very, happy day in my life.

Marriage

We have been married nearly three years. We have fulfilled our vows so far. It has been good. We can talk about anything; we don't have to agree with each other on every issue. We respect each other's differences and we rarely have arguments. We both give and we both receive. We are continually learning from each other. Wayne is very supportive of my recovery and the time it takes. He doesn't seem to have an addiction so he is still learning about them. (Hopefully, not how to get one.)

He goes to sleep much earlier than I do. Every night, I tuck him in and we will snuggle for a few minutes. Then, he tells me three things he loves about me and I tell him three things I love about him. I have to pay attention to what he does for me during the day so I will have three things. I need to do nice things for him so he will have something to love about me. "I love you because you bring me flowers. I love you because you are fun to be with. I love you because you are a good man."

We love dancing together. We try to go dancing every week for an hour or two. We do Country Western Progressive, Waltz, Three-Step, East Coast Swing, West Coast Swing, Cha-Cha, and a little Line Dancing. We take lessons whenever we can to continually improve our skills.

We enjoy traveling together, playing Bridge with close friends, playing games, walking, watching movies, laughing, being silly, and especially, spending time with our families. Heck, we even enjoy grocery shopping. My kids love Wayne and his love me. All our children and their spouses get along well with each other. When we are together, it is very loud. We have perfected talking and listening at the same time in our family: no ones takes turns. We have so much fun!

Life Today

I can exercise. I can walk for hours. I dance for 6 hours

on Dance Seminar Saturday. I can go to a water park in a swimming suit. I can snorkel. I can laugh. I can drive in England. (Alright, my son will say, "Not very well.") I can get around on foot, on trains and public transportation in Italy without knowing the language. (Yes, Mekala, I did get us lost a few times, but we finally found our way.) I had the courage to drive 22 hours with Myka to Guadalajara, Mexico and leave her there to live her life. I can learn continually. (I do have an insatiable desire to learn about so many things.) I can do silly things such as wearing my tiara to the grocery store with my daughters. I can hug. I can feel many different emotions besides fear. I can express displeasure. I can tell people I love them. I can enjoy beautiful sunsets, walks down the beach, full moons and fresh flowers. I feel I am living life to its fullest.

At one point in my life, I was afraid I would wake up when I was 80 years old and regret all the things I didn't do. Today I know I will not be able to fit in all the things I want to do. It seems unbelievable that I used to wake up dreading living another day! I think I had bad decades before program. Now, I never have a bad day. Oh, I sometimes have shitty minutes and every once in a while an hour stinks, but never a bad day. I have been abstinent. I prayed and did my writings and my gratitude list. When those are in my plus column, it is a pretty good day.

I continue working on my recovery because I don't think I will ever graduate. I go to my meetings. I believe if "I keep doing what I'm doing, I will keep getting what I'm getting." That is not a bad deal, because it brings me much happiness and a better understanding of myself. I have the fruits of my labor in the form of healthy relationships and a very happy, satisfying life. Life continues to get better all the time. I can't wait to see what else God has in store for me!

When I think about the lessons I have learned from skinned knees and elbows, of what I was like before I began my recovery, I am amazed. I am a miracle. My life is so sweet.

I hope you will find some help for your overeating issues in the 500 Solutions. If I can recover, so can you. If I can do it, you can do it. You, too, are a miracle waiting to happen. I hope and pray you don't miss life and the true happiness you can get from working the steps and working with other compulsive overeaters.

[1]_Alcoholics Anonymous_, Alcoholics Anonymous World Services. Inc. ©1976

[2]_Twelve Steps and Twelve Traditions_, Alcoholics Anonymous World Services, Inc. ©1953, Sixteenth printing 1978.

[3]_Alcoholics Anonymous_, ©1976, pages 285-286.

[4]_Twelve Steps and Twelve Traditions_, page 76.

[5]_Alcoholics Anonymous_, ©1976, pages 83-84.

[6]Ibid, page 76.

[7]_Alcoholics Anonymous_, ©1976, pages 60-61.

[8]"Nutrition Action Health Letter", Center for Science in the Public Interest, April 1999, p. 8.

[9]_Alcoholics Anonymous_, ©1976, pages 132-133.

[10]Alanon Family Groups. "Just For Today" Card.

[11] _Alcoholics Anonymous_, ©1976, page 449.

Chapter Two

Your Dream and Commitment

I suggest you get a notebook (It doesn't need to be pretty or fancy) to write your journey through the following Solutions. There will be numerous writing assignments.

Now write down what you would like your life to look like. Write your dreams and don't be afraid to dream big.

I want_____ physically.

I want_____ emotionally.

I want _____ socially.

I want_____ spiritually.

I want_____ materially.

I want_____ mentally.

I want_____ sexually.

Please think about what you are willing to commit to do to recover from overeating. Please write your commitment.

I commit to do (physical) _____.

I commit to do (emotional)_____.

I commit to do (social) _____.

I commit to do (spiritual) _____.

I commit to do (material) _____.

I commit to do (mental) _____.

I commit to do (sexual) _____.

Chapter Three

500 Solutions

The following list of 500 Solutions are things you can do instead of overeat. There is no magic. However, I believe if you think and write about these, you will be too busy to overeat! They are all just suggestions and not a particular dogma of mine. Seriously, these are some of the many ideas and concepts that I have examined and so have many others in many recovery rooms. None of these are totally my own creative ideas. They are a synthesis of many years of working my program. There is no specific order to work them. You can do them in order or you can just randomly open the book. I suggest you take those that sound like something you need to address and work those first. Your recovery will be the result of working the Twelve-Steps.

If there are suggestions that illicit a reaction of "No way, I'm not doing that, it's too stupid," circle it and come back to it later. I recommend you examine your hesitancy to take that action. Pay close attention to what your instincts are telling you.

If you don't try all of the suggestions, can you honestly say that the 500 Solutions or the Twelve-Steps don't work? Will you always wonder what would have happened if you had tried them?

I heard somewhere many years ago that we need to do action on what information we have before we seek more information. Always looking for "THE ANSWER" can be a way to avoid working on the answers we do have today.

I know you want to recover and I want you to recover, too. I don't want anyone else to die from this disease.

1. Go to your medical doctor and get a complete physical and discuss your plan to lose weight.

2. Write about your feelings about seeing your medical doctor.

3. Write down your top weight.

4. Write your feelings about that weight.

5. Write down today's weight.

6. Write your feelings about today's weight.

7. Write down your goal weight.

8. Write your feelings about your goal weight.

9. Close your eyes and imagine going to a party of your choice at your goal weight.

   - How would you be dressed?
   - What would you be doing at the party?
   - Who is at the party?

10. Write your reaction to the party – use as much detail as possible.

11. Close your eyes and imagine going to a party of your choice at today's weight.

    - How would you be dressed?
    - What would you be doing at the party?
    - Who is at the party?

12. Write your reaction to the party – use as much detail as possible.

13. Close your eyes and imagine going to a party of your choice weighing 50-100 pounds more than your weight today.

   - How would you be dressed?
   - What would you be doing at the party?
   - Who is at the party?

14. Write your reaction to the party – use as much detail as possible.

15. Go to see a registered dietician. (Many people claim to be nutritionists, but have little training. Check out their qualifications.)

16. Write about your feelings about the dietician's plan.

17. Research low-fat diets.

18. Write about your feelings about low-fat diets.

19. Research low-carb diets.

20. Write about your feelings about low-carb diets.

21. Research "basic four food group" diets.

22. Write about your feelings about "basic four food group" diets.

23. Research the food pyramid diets.

24. Write about your feelings about food pyramid diets.

25. Research 1200 – 1500 calorie diets.

26. Write about your feelings about counting calories.

27. Research diabetic exchange diets.

28. Write about your feelings about diabetic exchange diets.

29. Research the American Heart Association diet.

30. Write about your feelings about the American Heart Association diet.

31. Go to a Weight Watchers® meeting.

32. Write about your feelings of the Weight Watchers® food plan.

33. Research any other food plans.

34. What food plan sounds the most nutritious to you?

35. What food plan do you think better suits you?

36. Write on your willingness to go to any length to recover.

37. Write down your top 10 excuses.

38. Write how you can change those excuses into actions.

39. Write a history of your eating behaviors.

40. Write a list of diets you have tried?

41. Write a list of other methods you tried to lose weight.

42. Write a list of things you "think" might work to lose weight.

43. What has prevented you from trying those things?

44. What do you estimate you spent on binge foods yesterday?

45. What do you estimate you spent on binge foods last week?

46. What do you estimate you spent on binge foods last month?

47. What do you estimate you spent on binge foods last year?

48. How much have you spent to lose weight this month?

49. How much have you spent to lose weight this year?

50. List ten things you would do if you weren't overweight.

51. List ten things in your life that you would like to change.

52. List the people in your life you would like to change.

53. List the things in your life that are unacceptable to you.

54. Write an honest appraisal of how well you manage your life.

55. List the qualities you think people would use to describe you.

56. List the qualities describing your exterior self.

57. List the qualities describing your inner self.

58. List the qualities you would like to describe your exterior self.

59. List the qualities you would like to describe your inner self.

60. Write all the things your being overweight has cost you emotionally.

61. Write all the things your being overweight has cost you physically.

62. Write all the things your being overweight has cost you materially.

63. Write all the things your being overweight has cost you socially.

64. Write all the things your being overweight has cost you spiritually.

65. Write a letter to the "normal weight" self inside of you. Tell him/her about your fears.

66. Write a letter to the "overweight self" inside of you. Tell him/her about your fears

67. Write a gratitude letter to your overweight body for the gifts it has given you, ways it has protected you.

68. Write letter to your overweight body about your anger of being fat.

69. Write letter expressing your sadness of having been overweight.

70. Write a letter about the shame you have felt about your weight.

71. Write about your embarrassment about your body.

72. Write about your feelings about your sexuality and your body.

73. Write about the possibility of using your fat for sexual protection.

74. Write about the possibility of using your fat as a physical barrier to keep others away.

75. List 10 excuses your weight provides for not doing things you don't want to do.

76. List 10 excuses your weight provides for not doing things you do want to do.

77. Write how you think your partner feels about your weight.

78. Write how you think your partner would feel about you at goal weight.

79. Write how you think your friends feel about your weight.

80. Write how you think your friends would feel about you at goal weight.

81. Write how you think your family feels about your weight.

82. Write how you feel your family would feel about you at goal weight.

83. Write how you feel about your weight after working on these Solutions so far..

84. Write how you think you would feel about yourself at goal weight after working these Solutions.

85. Every time you want to binge this week, figure the cost and send that amount to the local food pantry for homeless people.

86. Every time you want to binge this week, figure the cost and save it until you can afford a body massage.

87. Does your weight prevent you from getting body massages? Write about it.

88. Do you think your boss or co-workers would treat you differently than if you were thin?

89. Go to at six least Overeaters Anonymous (OA) meetings.

90. If you don't like that meeting, go to another.

91. If you don't like that meeting, go to another one.

92. If you don't like that one, call the World Service Office (www.oa.org) and get information about starting a new meeting.

93. Buy the Twelve-Step literature of Overeaters Anonymous.

94. Buy the literature of Alcoholics Anonymous (AA).

95. Read the OA literature with an open mind.

96. Read the AA literature and substitute the words, compulsive overeater for alcoholic.

97. Read any Twelve-Step Program's literature and do the word substitution.

98. Read the literature as a textbook, not a novel about other people's lives.

99. Make notes when you identify with what you read in Program literature.

76

100. Make a list of all the judgmental statements you have had about the 500 Solutions.

101. Make a list of all the judgmental statements you have had about the literature you are reading.

102. Write down every critical thought you have today about yourself.

103. Write down every critical thought you have today about others.

104. Write down every nice thought you have about yourself today.

105. Write down every nice thought you have about others today.

106. Look a mirror, into your eyes and tell yourself, "I love you." Can you do it?

107. Practice looking yourself in the eyes everyday and saying it until you believe it.

108. Write your definition of a good friend.

109. Would you qualify as a good friend to others? If so, why? If not, why?

110. Write on "Do I treat myself as well as I would a friend?"

111. Read, study, and ask questions about sponsorship within the Twelve-Step Programs.

112. Write down what qualities you are looking for in a sponsor.

113. Ask someone at OA to sponsor you.

114. Call your sponsor.

115. Ask yourself, "Am I worthy of having a sponsor and the time they will invest in my recovery?" Write about it.

116. Ask yourself, "Am I worthy of recovery and the time I will invest in my recovery?" Write about it.

117. Ask your sponsor how to get started working the steps.

118. Discuss your food plan with your sponsor.

119. Begin to commit your daily food plan to your sponsor by telephone or email.

120. Do not lie to your sponsor. Write on why that is important.

121. Write all synonyms you can for the word **love.** (I can come up with two possible ones.)

122. Write all synonyms for **lying**. (I can come up with about seventy-five.)

123. Write the reasons you think for the difference in the numbers of the two.

124. Read Step One in OA and AA literature.

125. Work Step One and share your work with a sponsor.

126. Read Step Two in OA and AA literature.

127. Discuss Step Two with your sponsor.

128. Often heard at meetings, "Came, Came to, Came to believe." Write what that means to you.

129. Work Step Two and share your work with a sponsor.

130. Read Step Three in OA/AA literature.

132. Look up the definitions of 'care' and 'protection'.

133. Write about your willpower in all areas except food.

134. Write about your willpower in the area of food.

135. Talk to the newcomers at the OA meeting.

136. Call at least one OA member besides your sponsor every day.

137. Find online meetings to support your face-to-face OA meetings. (Not substitute)

138. Join or start an OA Internet "Loop" of Recovery.

139. Buy a Program-related meditation book.

140. Read a Program meditation book everyday.

141. Ask yourself if you are ready to do Step Three. Write about your reservations and fears in making that decision.

142. Write a "want ad" for the God you would want in your life.

143. Work your Third Step with your sponsor.

144. Share your recovery at a meeting. (You have no personality until you start to share. People won't know you. Everyone in the room was scared, to some degree, the first time they shared.)

145. Do it scared. Write about that concept.

146. Write about your concept of a Higher Power before age seven.

147. Write about your belief about a Higher Power after age 7 until early adulthood.

148. List ten negative thoughts you have about God.

149. Write about the people who helped you form those thoughts about God.

150. Who influenced your beliefs about who or what God is or is not?

151. How is your concept of your God like your father or father figure?

152. How is your concept of your God different from your father or father figure?

152. How is your personality and your idea of God the same?

153. How is your personality different from what your idea of God is?

154. Put on some soft music.

155. Relax.

156. Take 10 deep breaths.

157. Imagine walking through a forest.

158. Imagine going to a safe place.

159. Image the smells, the feel, the color, the texture, and the sounds of your safe place.

160. Are you indoors or outdoors in your safe place?

161. Once you have the image of your safe place, imagine your Higher Power coming to you.

162. Is your HP a grandfather with white robes, a young Jesus, a grandmother, a small inner child, a bright light, a warmth, an androgynous being, an animal or what else do you imagine?

163. Tell your Higher Power about your anger, pain, fear, guilt and love.

164. Write a letter to yourself from your God. Don't try to think about it, just write whatever comes to you.

165. Share your letter with a friend or your sponsor.

166. Write about your safe place.

167. Write about your experience doing the above exercise.

168. What are your positive and negative thoughts about it?

169. Spend some time outdoors.

170. Try to notice all the details of the outdoors; the smell, the sounds, the temperature, and the colors you see.

171. Try to be 100% present when you are somewhere. Try to stop your mind for a moment.

172. Do the first three steps every morning.

173. Write about fear and how it has paralyzed your life.

174. Ask yourself how you can do a "fearless moral inventory"? Why is that mentioned in the Step?

175. Read Step Four in the OA/AA literature.

176. Find a fourth step guidebook. Read it.

177. Decide what method you want to use.

178. Discuss your method of the Fourth Step you have chosen to use.

179. Make a commitment on a date to have your Fourth Step completed.

180. Start writing it.

181. Write on perfectionism and how it affects your life today.

182. Ask your sponsor for assistance if you have something in your inventory that there isn't a word to describe.

183. Decide if you want to do the Fifth Step with your sponsor.

184. Keep your commitment to write your Fourth Step.

185. Are you writing everything? Is it something important enough to be included in it? I heard, "If it is important enough to remember, put it in."

186. Put the good things about yourself in your inventory also.

187. Consider doing some needlework. It's hard to needlepoint and eat cheese puffs at the same time.

188. Buy fresh vegetables, i.e. purple cabbage, celery, carrots, green peppers, once a week to go in your salad. Cut them up and place them in a plastic bowl. Add a handful to fresh lettuce or spinach and you have a great salad. It is so convenient and quick when mealtime comes.

189. Cook extra protein and vegetables and freeze to make your own frozen dinners to have on days you don't have time to cook.

190. Have a Plan B in case Plan A doesn't work. Discuss these with your sponsor in advance. There will be times when we can't follow our Plan A.

191. Make a list of your favorite restaurants and plan a meal you can eat when you go there.

192. Write about the difference between deprivation and freedom in regards to food.

193. Make a list of foods you think are the most problematic to you.

194. Write what feelings you have when you think of giving them up.

195. Make a list of the ones you are willing to let go today.

196. Make a list of the ones you are not willing to say goodbye to yet.

197. Write about "willingness".

198. Write on the concept "You don't have to be willing, you just have to do it".

199. Write on the areas of your life where you are the most rebellious.

200. Read the Fifth Step in the OA/AA literature.

201. Ask someone to hear your Fifth Step. This may or may not be your sponsor.

202. With the person who hears your inventory, make a list of your character defects.

203. Make a list of 25 things you would do if you weren't afraid.

204. Decide if you want to hold on to your resentments any longer. If so, how long?

205. Read Step 6 in the OA/AA literature.

206. Write on the benefits that your character defects bring to your life, i.e. when I put others down, I get to feel better than.

207. Read Step 7 in the OA/AA literature.

208. Decide if you want to hold on to your fears any longer. If so, how long?

209. Humbly ask God to remove your shortcomings, if and when you are ready.

210. Read Step 8 in the OA/AA literature.

211. Make a list of the people to whom you need to make amends.

212. Divide your list into the people you want to do amends to now, in the future, never.

213. Date your list for future reference.

214. Discuss your amends you are going to make with your sponsor and pray about them. (You might be surprised when people on your future list re-enter your life.)

215. Read something spiritual, anything.

216. See a personal trainer.

217. Join a gym.

218. Buy fresh pineapple. It is cheaper than a half-gallon of ice cream.

219. Freeze grapes for a healthy snack.

220. Take a dance class.

- Ballroom
- Country Western
- Tap
- Jazz
- Line Dancing
- Square
- Contra
- Swing
- Folk

221. Write on your feelings about taking dance classes.

222. Take a water aerobics class.

223. Take an aerobic dance class.

224. Contact a friend to walk with you.

225. Join a Walking club.

226. Lift bottles of water if you can't afford a class or gym.

227. Write about your experiences in gym class when you were at school.

228. Were you the last to be picked or the first when teams were chosen in P.E?

229. What were your feelings about your place?

230. Go rollerblading.

231. Ride a bicycle.

232. Walk the stairs at lunch.

233. Park in the farthest parking spot from the door.

234. Take a quick walk at lunch. It all adds up.

235. Buy an exercise video. (Or use the one in your cabinet that you already own.)

236. Take swimming lessons.

237. Look at yourself in the mirror today and tell yourself, "I love you." Is it getting any easier?

238. Invite your friends over for an evening and ask them to bring magazines.

239. Serve only non-caloric beverages or tell friends to BYOB.

240. You and your friends look through magazines and cut out any word, phrase or picture of what you want in your lives.

241. Plan A: Make a visual poster of what want.

242. Look at your poster everyday.

243. Plan B: Sort your words, pictures and phrases into categories of what you want.

  - Spiritually
  - Physically
  - Emotionally
  - Friends
  - Family
  - Relationships
  - Internal Qualities
  - Financially
  - Travel
  - Home
  - Garden
  - Your dreams

244. Make a collage of your items in a large photo book.

245. Look at your book often.

246. Go to an extra meeting today.

247. Avoid reading the paper or watching the news for one week.

248. Did the world make it without your knowing what was going on in the news?

249. Write about your feelings during and after the "no news" week. Was it hard?

250. Write about your opinion of overeating being an addiction.

251. Read Step 9 in the OA/AA literature.

252. Make a direct amend.

253. Write about your reactions to the amends process.

254. Go for a walk, even if it is around the room.

255. Go for another walk, longer this time.

256. Move your body, somehow somewhere.

257. Buy fresh blueberries in season.

258. Wash and freeze blueberries individually on a cookie sheet. When frozen, bag in one-cup servings. Eat them frozen.

259. Start a "Seeing God's Miracles in My Life" list. Look for synchronicity in occurrences. Continue to add to it as you go through your recovery.

260. Write on what your rebellion gets you in life.

261. Smile and nod at speakers in meetings, it is a great service.

262. Come early and help set up chairs at the meeting.

263. Stay late and help put up chairs.

264. Go to an OA workshop.

265. Go to an open AA meeting.

266. Go to an OA retreat.

267. Write about how your weight affects your partner.

268. Write about how your weight affects your children, if you have them.

269. Write about how your weight affects your family.

270. Write about any shame you have about your weight.

271. Write about your body image.

272. Go to an OA convention.

274. Chair an OA meeting.

275. Write about your reactions to your weight loss.

276. Write about "Other people's opinions of me are none of my business?"

277. Write about how easy it is for you to say "No."

278. Write about the physical limitations your weight causes you.

279. Start looking at the style of clothes you want to wear.

280. Write what messages (spoken or unspoken) your father gave you about your body as a child.

281. Write what messages (spoken or unspoken) your mother gave you about your body as a child.

282. Write what messages (spoken or unspoken) your father gave you about your body as a teenager.

283. Write what messages (spoken or unspoken) your mother gave you about your body as a teenager.

284. Write what messages (spoken or unspoken) your father gave you about your body as an adult.

285. Write what messages (spoken or unspoken) your mother gave you about your body as an adult.

286. What are the messages you have received from the media about body sizes?

287. What is the most embarrassing thing that anyone ever said about your weight?

288. Write what messages (spoken or unspoken) your siblings gave you about your body as a child.

289. Write what messages (spoken or unspoken) your siblings gave you about your body as a teenager.

290. Write what messages (spoken or unspoken) your siblings gave you about your body as an adult.

291. What messages did you receive about gender in your family of origin?

292. What are the disadvantages of being male/female?

293. What are the advantages of being male/female?

On a scale of one to ten, how would you rate your life before program in the area of:

294. Physical. Explain.

295. Spiritual. Explain.

296. Emotional. Explain.

297. Mental. Explain.

298. Sexual. Explain.

On a scale of one to ten, how would you rate your life today after working the 500 Solutions and the Steps in the area of:

299. Physical. Explain.

300. Spiritual. Explain.

301. Emotional. Explain.

302. Mental. Explain.

303. Sexual. Explain.

304. Volunteer to give service at the Intergroup level of your area.

305. Read the Twelve Traditions in the OA/AA literature.

306. Write how the Traditions can be applied to your personal life.

307. Read the Tenth Step in OA/AA literature.

308. Do you owe an amends to anyone for your behavior today?

The Big Book says to watch the following:

309. Selfishness – How did you do today?

310. Dishonesty – How well did you do?

311. Resentment – How about this area?

312. Fear – How much time did I give it?

313. Ask yourself these questions every day.

314. Write a letter to your HP about your feelings today.

315. When something upsetting happens, ask yourself "How much do I have to eat to change what happened?"

316. When disturbed by something, use the "Two Year Test" – Ask yourself, "How important is this going to be in two years?"

317. Write about the statement "Yesterday is history."

318. Write about the statement "Tomorrow is a mystery."

319. Write about the statement "Today is a gift, that is why it is called a present."

320. Look at all the things you tried to control.

321. Write about other's reactions to your attempts to control today.

322. Read Step Eleven in the OA/AA literature.

323. Write your reactions to what you read.

324. Write about what prayer means to you.

325. Write about the different types of meditation you have tried.

326. Research meditation on the Internet.

327. Buy a meditation CD.

328. How many minutes do you commit to mediate today?

329. How many times do you commit to mediate this week?

330. Talk to your sponsor about your commitment.

331. Are you sponsoring? If not, why not?

332. List five reasons you are not sponsoring.

333. Tell the truth about your reasons. Are they really just excuses, selfishness, or fear?

334. If you are sponsoring, write about the benefits to your program have you received?

335. Write about your frustrations about being a sponsor.

336. Are you still calling your sponsor? If not, write your reasons.

337. Tell the truth about your reasons. Are they really just excuses? Write about it.

338. Write about you fears of success.

339. Write about your fears of failure.

340. Write about your weight loss and how it feels today.

341. Look at yourself in the mirror and say, "I love you." How does that feel today?

342. What does "conscious contact" mean to you?

343. What does the part of the Eleventh Step "Praying only for the knowledge of His will and the power to carry it out" mean to you?

344. How does that statement fit into your beliefs about prayer?

345. What is the difference between spiritual and religious to you?

346. Write about the prejudices you have about religion.

347. Write about the differences in the religion of your youth and yours today, if you have one.

348. If you have no religion today, write about it.

349. Find the Third, Seventh and Eleventh Step prayers in the Big Book.

350. Memorize those prayers.

351. Write about your feelings about the word "prayer".

352. Write your feelings about the idea of praying for God's Will and praying for specifics.

353. How have your beliefs about a Higher Power changed since working the 500 Solutions and the Twelve-Steps?

354. Write on the concept of "Act as if".

355. Write on the idea, "Faith is the opposite of fear".

356. Write on the slogan, "Nothing tastes as good as abstinence feels".

357. Write on the slogan, "Easy does it".

358. Write on the slogan, "Fear is false evidence appearing real."

359. Write on the slogan, "Fake it until you make it."

360. Write on the slogan, "Abstinence is the most important thing in my life without exception."

361. Write on the saying, "When something else becomes more important than your abstinence, it is the second thing you are going to lose."

362. Write about the saying, "I fit my lifestyle into my recovery instead of fitting my recovery into my lifestyle."

363. Write a list of the food you are having the most difficulty with in your food plan.

364. Eat your meal before you go to parties.

365. Call your host before going to dinner parties to find out the menu and take foods to supplement your needs.

366. Focus on the people at the party instead of the food.

367. When someone keeps trying to get you to eat something, it is okay to ask him/her, "Why is it so important to you that I eat it?"

368. Write about the saying, "One bite may not hurt but what will it do to help?"

369. Write about the saying, "One bite is too many and a thousand are not enough."

370. If it is on your food plan, make a pumpkin pie with the recipe on the can of pumpkin using Splenda®, non-fat evaporated milk and no crust.

371. Make dips with non-fat yogurt for your fresh vegetables.

372. Take a plastic bag with a serving of baked corn chips with you to Mexican restaurants.

373. Buy fresh flowers with the money you saved from not having a binge.

374. Bake an apple with cinnamon and artificial sweetener of choice in the microwave.

375. Start paying attention to determine who tries to sabotage your food plan.

376. Read the promises in the Big Book on page 83-84.

377. Which ones have you begun to experience?

378. Write about the statement from the Big Book, "Love and tolerance of others is our code."

379. Write about the statement from the Big Book, "What we really have is a daily reprieve contingent on the maintenance of our fit spiritual condition."

380. Write about the statement from the Big Book, "We are neither cocky nor or we afraid."

381. Read page 101 in the Big Book, which discusses whether we need to avoid places of temptation.

382. Write about your reaction to that reading.

383. Write about the idea of "not fondling food" in your mind.

384. Write a "nightmare of your later eating".

385. Write how you felt after your worst binge.

386. Write about the lengths that you are willing to go to recover today versus when you began the 500 Solutions.

387. Donate a copy of OA/AA literature to the public library.

388. Order a subscription of "Lifeline", the monthly magazine of Overeaters Anonymous.

389. Order a copy of "Lifeline" for your doctor's office.

390. Take action to take a meeting to the local jail or prison.

391. Send "To the Professional" pamphlets to the local therapists and physicians in your area.

392. Volunteer to answer the telephone for OA in your area.

393. Read about anonymity in OA/AA literature.

394. Contact a local newspaper about doing a public interest story about OA.

395. Suggest to your group to hold a "Family and Public Information Night".

396. Invite the local media to the "Family and Public Information Night" and give them information about the anonymity statement.

397. Write about what personal anonymity means to you and your group members.

398. Write an article to the "Lifeline" magazine.

399. Share your program with people who ask you how you have lost weight.

400. Contact school counselors about OA.

401. Start a new meeting.

402. Visit other meetings.

403. Invite guest speakers to tell their story at your meeting.

404. Start a formal Step Study group.

405. Go to coffee after the meeting with OA members.

406. Invite the newcomers to come to coffee.

407. Give service above the group level.

408. Become a delegate to attend regional assemblies.

409. Serve on committees at the regional level.

410. Serve as a delegate at the World Service level of OA.

411. Be an active member of a committee at the World Service Business Conference.

412. Make telephone calls to other members.

413. Share your "strength, hope, and experience" at meetings.

414. "Suit up and show up" at meetings.

415. Attend OA meetings in other cities when out of town.

416. Attend a retreat or convention in another city. (You have saved enough money from not overeating; you can afford it.)

There is a principle for every step. Write about each principle and how you feel it relates to the step.

417. Step One –   Honesty

418. Step Two –   Hope

419. Step Three –   Faith

420. Step Four –   Courage

421. Step Five –   Integrity

422. Step Six –   Willingness

423. Step Seven –   Humility

424. Step Eight –   Self-discipline

425. Step Nine –   Love

426. Step Ten –   Perseverance

427. Step Eleven –   Spiritual Awareness

428. Step Twelve –   Service

429. Write about the change in the level of trust you have *for* others since working your recovery program.

430. Write about the change in the level of trust you have *from* others since working your recovery program.

431. Write about the change in the level of trust you have for yourself since working your recovery program.

432. Write about your feelings about Tradition One – How your "personal recovery depends on OA unity."

433. How has your tolerance of other's opinions and beliefs changed?

434. Do you have the only requirement for membership - a desire to stop eating compulsively?

435. Do you honestly want to stop compulsively overeating or just to lose weight and keep it off? Write about that statement.

436. Do you include newcomers in your "circle" at meetings? Write about it.

437. Is there some service you feel you can do for OA that you are not doing?

438. Why not? Write about it exploring the reasons.

439. Are you self-supporting in your group? In money and service? Do you expect others to do it? Write about it.

440. Are you resentful of all the times I have suggested writing about things?

441. Write about your willingness today versus before reading this book.

442. What is the difference in "miracles versus magic"? Write about your beliefs.

443. Write about any remaining fears you may have today you want to release.

444. Read more of the OA/AA literature – there are many different books and pamphlets.

445. Read literature on co-dependency and look at the symptoms. Do you relate?

446. Look at yourself in the mirror today – Can you honestly say, "I love you"? Does it feel different from when you first started working your program?

447. Look up the definition of humility and write about it.

448. Write about any areas of shame that remains in your life.

449. Can you see "how your experiences can benefit others"?

450. Write about your money management since beginning your program.

451. Most of us spend the first money we ever receive on food. Write about any spending problems you may have had.

452. Our homes reflect our recovery. The messier the external – the messier the internal. Write how this relates to your home.

453. Write about any changes in your primary relationships since your recovery began.

454. Write what your values are in your life today.

455. If you knew your house would be destroyed in fifteen minutes, what things would you take out? (Excluding people or pets.)

456. What do those things represent to you? Write about them.

There are other addictions that can cause problems. Honestly rate the following on a level of 1 to 10 (one being the least and ten the highest). These can be used to avoid feelings or "living our lives."

457. Alcohol

458. Sugar

459. Television

460. Romance Novels

461. Being "Right"

462. Sex

463. Pornography

464. Caffeine

465. Computer games

466. Chat rooms

467. Cybersex

468. Prescription pills

469. Over-the-counter medications

470. Sleep

471. Movies

472. Illegal drugs

473. Religion

474. Sports - watching

475. Sports – participating

476. Relationships

477. Co-dependency

478. Emotional incest with children

479. Controlling others

480. Dependency on others

481. Write on any area you rated above four.

482. Write about any anger you felt about the list.

483. Write a letter expressing your anger about any of the solutions.

484. Write a list of the 10 most beneficial solutions for you.

485. Tell your loved ones three things you love about them today.

486. Ask three people what they love the most about you.

487. Use the question "What would the loving person do today in this situation?"

488. Write how you feel about Abraham Lincoln's statement, "When I do good I feel good, when I do bad I feel bad, and that's my religion."

489. Go to the beginning of the list of 500 solutions and see if your answers have changed since you began.

490. Write a sample day in your life today. Has it changed? Write about it.

491 What new goals do you have in your life?

492. Re-read Your Commitment and Dreams

493. Are your dreams bigger? Describe.

494. What are you doing today to work Steps 10-12?

495. Do you have any areas of your life you still need to write an inventory on?

496. How has your relationship with your Higher Power changed?

497. How can you "carry the message" today?

498. How have your self-esteem and self-confidence changed? Write about it.

499. As heard in program rooms all around the world, "Pass it on."

500. Live your life and live it fully to the best of your ability, today and always.

Remember,

500 Excuses

or

500 Solutions

YOUR CHOICE.

Comments can be sent to:
Tonna@overeating500Solutions.com

YOUR SOLUTIONS

1. _____

2. _____

3. _____

4. _____

5. _____

6. _____

7. _____

8. _____

9. _____

10. _____

11. _____

12. _____

13. _____

14. _____

15. _____

16. _____

17. _____

18. _____

19. _____

20. _____

21. _____

22. _____

23. _____

24. _____

25. _____

26. _____

27. _____

28. _____

29. _____

30. _____

31. _____

32. _____

33. _____

34. _____

35. _____

36. _____

37. _____

38. _____

39. _____

40. _____

41. _____

42. _____

43. _____

44. _____

45. _____

46. _____

47. _____

48. _____

49. _____

50. _____

51. _____

52. _____

53. _____

54. _____

55. _____

56. _____

57. _____

58. _____

59. _____

60. _____

61. _____

62. _____

63. _____

64. _____

65. _____

66. _____

67. _____

68. _____

69. _____

70. _____

71. _____

72. _____

73. _____

74. _____

75. _____

76. _____

77. _____

78. _____

79. _____

80. _____

81. _____

82. _____

83. _____

84. _____

85. _____

86. _____

87. _____

88. _____

89. _____

90. _____

91. _____

92. _____

93. _____

94. _____

95. _____

96. _____

97. _____

98. _____

99. _____

100. _____

101. _____

Please use your notebook for any additional Solutions you have.

You can also post them at

www.Overeating500Solutions.com

Chapter Five

Your Journal

Your Journal

Your Journal

Your Journal

Your Journal

Your Journal

Your Journal

Your Journal

Your Journal

Your Journal

About the Author

Tonna Brock, M.Ed, MS, LPC is a graduate of Texas Woman's University. She has been working in the eating disorder recovery field for 17 years. In private practice, she was the Owner and Director of Sherman and McKinney Family Counseling Centers for 11 years. For three years, Tonna taught "The Survey of Eating Disorders" class at the Collin County Community College in their eating disorder counselor certification program.

For more than 20 years, Tonna has been the main speaker at meetings, luncheons, workshops, retreats, treatment centers, seminars and conventions in the United States and Canada. She was the producer and co-host of a radio program, "Roads to Recovery" for several years.

Tonna is currently producing "KickStart into Recovery Retreats", a weekend for overeaters to learn more about their disease and begin their lifelong recovery. She is also available for public speaking engagements on eating disorders and her "God as I understand Him" workshops.

Contact Information:

Tonna Brock, M.Ed, MS, LPC
P.O. Box 684
McKinney, Texas 75070

www.Overeating500Solutions.com